MW01268633

Dr. Sebi Diet

The Complete Nutritional Guide to Plant-Based Alkaline Diet.Cookbook with 83 Recipes to Detox your Body, Liver Cleansing, Reverse Diabetes, and High Blood Pressure.21 Days Meal Plan and Meal Prep for Rapid Weight Loss with Dr. Sebi's Diet.

[Dr. John Tortora]

ISBN:9798662910706

CONTENTS

Introduction

Alkaline diets include foods that maintain a ph-balance above 7. The ph-scale is used to assess if it is acidic or alkaline. Seven is neutral, and it is not acidic or alkaline. Everything over seven is known to be acidic; everything is below alkaline. Alkaline diets mention foods which are deemed alkaline or that do not produce acid in the body when digested and prescribe consuming such foods to people.

Many people claim that the way we live in a culture today is incredibly harmful to our wellbeing. They conclude that consuming highly acidic products affects the quality of cells and body fluids. Sadly, this evidence was not applied to clinically in several clinical studies, although there were a variety of individuals who attempted alkaline diets and recorded impressive health benefits.

Alkaline diets can give some of their health benefits: decreased vitality, weight control, lower dependency or no insulin reliance on patients with diabetes, no acid reflux, enhancement in their hair, nails, eyes, better moods for sleep, mental stability, candida symptoms relief and just to name a couple.

This diet reduces body contaminants and encourages general wellbeing. It will make you take a safer, better approach to food.

It will also raise the chances of other diseases. If you have to lose weight, it can motivate you to do it easily and reliably. This is related to improved strength and resilience that everyone requires.

There is more to the alkaline diet than meets the eye. A few lines of short sentences is not enough to detail everything you need to know about it. This is why in this book; we are going to take a closer look at some cogent points made by Dr. Sebi.

This guide presents recipes for a variety of meals including the different ingredients and the steps involved in the preparation of the meal. This way, you will always have a variety of foods to pick from for every meal, spend less time brainstorming on what to eat and make it easier to adhere to the alkaline healthy living lifestyle.

Chapter 1: What is Dr. Sebi's Diet?

Doctor Sebi (real name Alfredo Darrington Bowman) is a native Honduran herbalist, healer, and therapist. His diet approach revolves around natural alkaline, plant-based foods and herbs and avoiding intake of acidic foods that are dangerous to the body. Many adherents of Doctor Sebi diets and his herbal approach to healing testify to its efficacy over the conventional Western medicine approach. The diet also helps to teach and improve healthy living even to this day (even after his death).

He started a USHA Healing village in Honduras that focuses on providing healing to people and also teach how to like an alkaline lifestyle.

What Was the Diet Based On?

The diet came into existence when he declared that it could heal and revitalize the human body from different illnesses by inducing an alkaline environment inside the body and removing harmful substances. It instructs the person to eat a set of predetermined ingredients, which include fruits and vegetables and other vegetarian edibles only, with the addition of taking a hefty dose of supplements.

He believed that the diseases inside our body are caused by the buildup of mucus in different organs—like if the heart had a buildup of mucus, it leads to heart disease, and if it is in excess in the pancreas, it causes diabetes. He also claimed that diseases thrive in acidic environments and die in an alkaline environment. He said that the diet would restore the body's original healthy start if we strictly follow it and consume the mixtures/supplements that he originally made. The body will then be cleansed and detoxified of harmful substances. Natural foods mentioned in this diet are high in alkalinity, and it raises the body pH, so according to Alfredo's theories, they can heal the body by creating an alkaline environment internally.

The diet is made up of lists of different vegetables, fruits, seeds, grains, nuts, and oils, with no addition of animal-sourced food. That is why the diet can also be considered a vegan diet. However, it is even more restrictive than that as some vegetables, grains, and fruits are banned from being consumed. For example, you are not permitted to eat seedless fruits in this diet. Also, to get the maximum and continuous benefit, Dr. Sebi says to follow this diet for the entirety of your life, which makes the diet even more strict and restrictive.

As it is a popular diet, many people on social media have claimed this diet has helped them in healing, but there are no scientific studies present that can vouch for those claims.

Eating Naturally with Dr. Sebi's Teachings

The Dr. Sebi diet is often referred to as the African biomineral balance. This was how he would cure people of a variety of diseases. It is basically a vegan diet that is made up of foods that he called "electric" or alkaline foods. It is suggested that, while following this diet, you also take his healing supplements.

You cannot eat any meat or animal products while on this diet, as well as foods that contain a lot of starch. The reason for this is that you are only supposed to eat alkaline-forming foods, and those foods form acids.

Meat products cause uric acid production, dairy produces cause lactic acid, and starch causes carbonic acid. All of these acids will buildup, which causes a buildup of mucus. The mucus robs our cells of oxygen. However, if you eat electric foods, they feed the body. The human body is electrical, so it needs electric food to function.

This diet is made up of grains, teas, nuts, veggies, and fruits. Among the foods,you can eat are wild rice, amaranth, quinoa, mushrooms, watercress, kale, dates, figs, mangos, avocados, and much more. These foods will help to nourish your body and won't end up causing an accumulation of mucus.

If you plan on really starting this diet, you must make sure that you really want it. The first thing you will need to do is to make some changes to how you eat. You will probably find that this is going to require you to be your best emotional state and the right state of mind.

Eating is a big part of our life and the types of things we consume form strong habits that can end up lasting our entire life. It can be very hard to break these habits and deal with the influence of family and friends. That means, before you jump right into this diet, you should take some time thinking about changing how you eat. You don't want to promise yourself this and then end up not being able to follow through just because you weren't prepared.

Instead, you should begin slowly. You can even talk to your family and friends. The reaction you can get from people when you talk to them about Dr. Sebi's diet will vary. Some will want to learn more, while others will write it off as bunk.

That being said, you shouldn't tire yourself by trying to convince everybody else before you make sure that it is right for you. Your vitality, health improvements, and cleaner outlook will show your family way more than just your words.

Once you do start making the transition, the first thing you need to do is to start reading food ingredient labels on everything. This will help you to stay conscious about what you are drinking and eating. When you are first starting out, before you live completely by the nutritional guide, this awareness is going to provide you with the incentive to change things as you continue on. Later on, if you do end up straying from the diet, you will still be able to remain conscious about what you are eating.

If you have long been a meat-eater, that may be the hardest thing to transition from. The best thing you can do is to start making the transition from meats by switching to eating only fish. Then you can slowly start eating less and less fish each week.

It is also important that you start making your own snacks. This will ensure if you do get the urge to snack, that you will have good snacks to eat. Approved nuts and raisins are a good choice.

Then you need to make sure that you are eating all of the correct foods. That means you need to learn what foods are and aren't on the nutritional guide. You must stick to only those foods. At first, this will feel tough, and that is expected. In fact, it is very hard to do in our society when only the bad foods are pushed at us. This is the reason why I stressed that you must be emotionally ready.

You also need to make sure you are drinking plenty of water. While we have all known for a while now that water is a very important part of our health, most of us are still not drink enough. Plus, there are a lot of Dr. Sebi products that you will be taking, like the Bromide Plus Powder, contain herbs that act as diuretics. That means you have to take extra care to make sure you don't allow yourself to get dehydrated.

Tips to Get Started with the Dr. Sebi Diet

To follow Dr. Sebi's diet, you need to strictly adhere to his rules, which are present on his website. Here is a list of his guidelines below:

1. Do not eat or drink any product or ingredient not mentioned in the approved list for the diet. It is not recommended and should never be consumed when following the diet.

2. You have to drink almost one gallon (or more than three liters) of water every day. It is recommended to drink spring water.

 3. You have to take Dr. Sebi's mixtures or products one hour before consuming your medications.

 4. You can take any of Dr. Sebi's mixtures/products together without any worry.

 5. You need to follow the nutritional guidelines stringently and punctually take Dr. Sebi's mixtures/products daily.

6. You are not allowed to consume any animal-based food or hybrid products.

7. You are not allowed to consume alcohol or any kind of dairy product.

8. You are not allowed to consume wheat, only natural growing grains as listed in the nutritional guide

9. The grains mentioned in the nutritional guide can be available in different forms, like pasta and bread, in different health food stores. You can consume them.

10. Do not use fruits from cans; also, seedless fruits are not recommended for consumption.

11. You are not allowed to use a microwave to reheat your meals.

Chapter 2: Food Principles

As you may have noticed, the Dr. Sebi diet is not like any other. Where other diets either have a bunch of information that you can't figure out what it means, Dr. Sebi's diet is very straightforward. You have the food list that you have to stick with, you have the supplements that you should take, and then you have the rules we are going to go over. While the diet does require giving up a lot of stuff, it is very easy to see what you should and should not do, which, in the long run, makes it easier to follow. Let's take a look at the rules.

You are only allowed to eat the foods that are listed on the nutritional guide.

The nutritional guide is the only guide you have for this diet, and those foods are the only approved foods. It really can't get any more straightforward than that. The only things that aren't really listed on the nutritional guide that you do get to consume are herbs that are most often used in supplements. Any herb that is used in Dr. Sebi's supplements, you can use in other ways as well, such as sea moss, burdock, and bladderwrack. You won't find those things on the nutritional guide, but they can be consumed in various ways and not just through the supplements.

You have to consume a gallon of water each day.

That may sound like a lot, but with some planning, you can do it. Just so you know, a gallon of water comes out to 3.8 liters. Your body is made up of mostly water and it needs water to work properly. There are so many people walking around who are dehydrated and dehydration has the power to make you feel awful. Dehydration can cause you to faint, feel fatigued or irritable, look tired, breathe quickly, have a rapid heartbeat, feel dizzy, have dry skin, and so much more. While some of these only happen in severe cases of dehydration, like fainting, the other symptoms are so common that people don't even think anything about it.

If you are on medications, take your Dr. Sebi supplements an hour before you take your medications.

Dr. Sebi does not want you to stop taking medications if you are currently using them. They do serve a purpose in your body, for now. Once you have followed his diet for a while and gotten rid of the disease, you can stop taking your medications under the supervision of your doctor. This will make sure that you don't end up hurting yourself more. That said, if you are currently on medication for diabetes, high blood pressure, or what have you, you need to make sure that all of your Dr. Sebi supplements are taken an hour before you take those prescriptions.

You are not allowed to consume any type of animal products.

First off, we are the only mammals who feed their young milk from other mammals. Cows do not ask a goat for their milk to feed their babies. Then there is the act of eating meat. If you look at any carnivorous animals out there, such as lions, bears, or wolves, they all have sharp pointy canines and claws. Humans have small canine teeth and soft fingernails. Carnivores are provided the tools they need in order to tear flesh without the need for forks and knives. Their jaws also only move up and down, which gives them the ability to tear chunks of meat out of the prey.

You cannot consume alcohol.

Alcohol, as we all know, is very detrimental to our health, especially our liver. Alcohol is also very acidic. The liver has the hard job of breaking down harmful chemicals, and alcohol is only made up of harmful chemicals. When the liver has to work overtime in getting rid of alcohol, it can lead to cirrhosis, jaundice, and hepatitis. Alcohol is a waste product that the body wants to get, and the smallest amount affects the body. If you consume more alcohol than the body can process, you start to become intoxicated as it builds up. This will slow down how your body functions, including the immune system. This is why heavy drinkers are more likely to develop illnesses and it also increases their risk of several different types of cancer.

Do not use the microwave to cook your food because it will kill it.

Microwave ovens were made for convenience, and convenient they are, but they aren't really good for you or your food. Microwaves turn electricity into electromagnetic waves, which are called microwaves. This makes the molecules in your food vibrate and spin, which is what makes them hot. If you rub your hands together really fast, you will be doing, basically, the same thing. The microwave does produce a type of radiation, but there are a lot of protective factors on the microwave itself that keeps the radiation from reaching you, as long as the microwave is still in good condition.

You cannot consume seedless or canned fruits.

You've likely had both the seeded and seedless varieties of foods and probably can't even notice a difference. But seedless fruits are not okay. They aren't even able to reproduce. The process that fruits go through to make them seedless creates something that our bodies don't even recognize, so they aren't able to use them.

Canned fruits are another best. By canned fruits, I mean those in the metal cans at the grocery store and not foods that you can naturally at home. The canned fruits at the store often contain trace amounts of BPA, bisphenol-A. The leading cause of BPA exposure is through eating canned foods. BPA exposure can lead to male sexual dysfunction, type 2 diabetes, and heart disease.

You cannot consume coffee or sodas, only spring water, and herbal teas.

Coffee, while not innately bad for your body, is also not all that great for you either. The caffeine in coffee is addictive, which causes people to crave more caffeine. The more you drink, the higher your tolerance for it grows, and the more you need to get the high you are looking for. Somebody also finds that coffee hurts their stomach and digestive tract, and can also lead to heartburn and stomach ulcers. While it can be hard to give up coffee, it will be worth it in the long run because you will be allowing your natural energy to return without the need of the caffeine.

While coffee may have some redeeming properties, soda has none. Not even diet soda. This shouldn't come as a surprise to anybody, but soda is bad for you. They are jam packed full of sugar. All of this sugar does nothing for your body and will not help satiate hunger. What they do is lead to weight gain. All of this sugar will then be turned into fat in your liver. Table sugar and corn syrup contain glucose and fructose. Every cell in your body can metabolize the glucose, but fructose is only able to be metabolized in the liver. Sugary sodas are the easiest way to consume too much fructose. When you constantly drink sodas, the liver will become overloaded and will turn the fructose into fat. This can lead to nonalcoholic fatty liver disease.

Sodas are also the number one cause of type 2 diabetes. In one study performed across 175 countries, looked at the connection between diabetes and sugar consumption, found that a single can of soda increased a person's diabetes risk by 1.1%. There are also no nutrients whatsoever in soda, only sugar. It does not provide your body with anything that it can use. They also contain caffeine, which means that they are addictive. Add in the sugar, it becomes even more addictive than coffee. Sugar can cause dopamine release, which makes you feel happy. Thus, your brain equates soda to being happy.

Lastly, sodas are absolutely horrible for your dental health. The carbonic acid and phosphoric acid in the sodas create an acidic environment in your mouth, which causes your teeth to decay. While these acids are bad for your teeth, the sugar is more harmful. The sugar gives energy to the bad bacteria in your mouth. Not only is the acid eroding away at your enamel, but the bad bacteria are thriving, and this all writes disaster for your dental health.

Chapter 3: Benefits of Dr. Sebi Diet

Give protection to bone density and muscle mass

Taking minerals into your body system plays a significant role in maintaining and developing the bones in your body. Research has proved to the truth that the more alkaline-rich fruits and vegetables you take regularly, the better you get protected from experiencing reduced bone muscle and strength known as Sarcopenia. What an alkaline diet does when you take it is to help in balancing the ratios of the various minerals in the body necessary for the bone-building and the maintenance of a lean muscle mass. The minerals that an alkaline diet balances are Phosphate, Magnesium, and Calcium. Another benefit of an alkaline diet in this regard is the improvement in the production of vitamin D absorption and growth hormones which helps in further protecting the bones and fighting against many chronic diseases.

Reduce the risk of hypertension and stroke

Another great benefit of eating an alkaline diet is the reduction of the risk of stroke and hypertension and individual is prone to have. A typical alkaline diet has an anti-aging effect. A robust result of the anti-aging effects is that it drastically reduces inflammation and fosters the growth of hormone production. This has been verified to help in the improvement of cardiovascular health and giving the body defense against typical health challenges like hypertension, high cholesterol, stroke, kidney stones, and possible memory loss.

Reduce chronic pain and inflammation

There is a correlation between alkaline diets and a drastic reduction in levels of chronic pain. Chronic acidosis is dangerous to the human health system. It is the primary cause of headaches, chronic back pain, joint pain, inflammation, menstrual symptoms, and muscle spasms.

Cases abound that show the health benefits of alkaline diets suffering from chronic pains. A study conducted showed that there was a significant level of decrease in the pain experienced by patients suffering from chronic back pain when they were supplements containing alkaline daily for four weeks.

Weight loss

This diet was not made with weight loss in mind, but because it is extremely restrictive, you will see weight loss. Also, one of the main reasons that this diet is effective in reducing weight is that it makes people stop consuming Western foods, which are highly caloric, oily, and sugary.

Weight loss occurs when you eat less or equal amounts of calories that you can burn. If you follow this diet—which is low in sugar, fat, and processed foods—you can get your perfect body.

Improves kidney function

Acidic diets mostly affect the health of the kidneys and damages the layers inside the organ system. To promote kidney health, the pH of the urine mustn't be acidic. By consuming a lot of alkaline food and removing acidic foods from our daily routine, we can reach this pH in which our kidneys remain safe and healthy. Alkaline diets do not affect the pH of the blood, but it can significantly affect the urine. Drinking a lot of water alongside this diet can improve kidneys even more. If you're suffering from any chronic kidney disease, then you should know that this diet is not targeted for you. You can follow the diet after consulting your doctor first.

Reduces the risk of cancer

There are almost no significant studies that show that an alkaline diet leads to decreased cases of cancer. However, there have been studies that show that if a person were to eat less meat and increase their consumption of fresh fruits and vegetables, then that person is at a lower risk of cancer. Also, another study showed that having more vitamins, like vitamin C, in your diet can prevent cancer. Generally, eating more fruits and vegetables and consuming less high fatty and sugary foods leads to a reduction in developing cancer.

Reduces the risk of heart disease

Heart disease is the major cause of death in the world. It is mainly caused by eating lots of fat and oily foods, which results in the development of plaque and blockage of arteries. In this diet, the consumption of fats goes down significantly, decreasing the chances of developing heart disease.

It has also been shown that growth hormones are related to decreased rates of heart disease. An alkaline diet increases the levels of growth hormones, so, in turn, it decreases heart disease as well.

Reduces the risk of muscle degradation

When we grow old or stop using our muscles, we tend to increase muscle loss. However, there was a study conducted in 2013 showing that people who follow the alkaline diet could decrease muscle degradation. The diet is low in red meat, so there is a risk of decreasing muscle mass and strength.

Increases intestinal health

With the addition of whole grains, there is a list of nuts and seeds that you can eat on this diet. It contributes to an increase in fiber intake, which increases the health of small and large intestines. It helps manage regular bowel movements, which reduces the risk of developing many diseases.

Decreases the harmful effects of processed foods

Processed foods have been linked to increased sugar intake and fat content. They also contain lots of calories but have very low nutritional value. Many additives and preservatives that have no purpose in our body are eliminated from our diets if we strictly avoid processed foods.

It helps the brain

The growth hormone is not only related to a better heart condition but also helps manage the health of the mind. It is related to an increase in memory and cognition. Eating a healthy diet rich in fruits and vegetables leads to better brain functioning.

It may improve back pain

Alkaline minerals are related to the reduction of back pain, but whether alkaline foods provide the same results has yet to be determined. There is a decent chance that the diet has similar effects.

Decreases the level of inflammation

Diets rich in fresh fruits and vegetables show a great decrease in oxidative stress and inflammation. This leads to less discomfort and fewer diseases developing in our bodies.

Prevent deficiency in magnesium and increases vitamin absorption

Magnesium plays an essential role in the human body as an increase in its quantity is necessary for the proper functioning of all the enzymes and processes in the human body. Deficiency in magnesium content will result in headaches, anxiety, heart complications, muscle pains, and sleep troubles. Magnesium is also needed by the body in the activation of vitamin D and preventing Vitamin D deficiency, necessary for the functioning of the endocrine and overall body immunity.

Improving cancer protection and immune function

Minerals are needed by the body in disposing of waste or in oxygenating the body. But when there is a shortage of the required minerals in the cells, the body suffers. Vitamin absorption is zeroed off whenever there is a mineral loss in the body. Also, toxins and pathogens will pile up in the body thereby weakening the immune system. But with alkaline diets, that cannot happen as research has proved that the death of cancerous cells happens more in an alkaline body. Alkaline diets will help in decreasing inflammation and the possible risks associated with dangerous diseases such as cancer.

Help you in maintaining a healthy balanced weight

When you eat more of alkaline diets, you are not just limiting the acidic content in your body but also protecting your body from the risks associated with obesity. This is possible as alkaline diets decrease the levels of Leptin and inflammation which has a direct effect on your hunger and   fat-burning   capacities.

Chapter 4: Alkaline Diets Dr. Sebi's, Nutritional guide

Vegetables

Current list 2019 (previous and recently added)

Wild arugula (added)

Okra (added back after being removed)

Purslane (verdolaga) – (added)

Watercress – (added)

Izote – (previously existing)

kale (previously existing)

Lettuce – except iceberg (previously existing)

Mushrooms - except shitake (previously existing)

Nopales also known as mexican cactus (previously existing)

Olives and olive oil (previously existing)

Onions (previously existing)

Sea vegetables - dulse wakame nori aramehijiki/ (previously existing)

Squash (previously existing)

Tomato – plum and cherry (previously existing)

Tomatillo (previously existing)

Turnip greens (previously existing)

Zucchini (previously existing)

Fruits

Recently added

Prickly pear (cactus fruit) – (added)

Tamarind – (added)

Previously existing

Apples

Limes

 currants

Figs

Cantaloupe

Berries

Bananas

Cherries

Raisins –seeded

Soursops

Grapes –seeded

Soft jelly coconuts / coconut oil

Papayas

Prunes

Melons –seeded

Mango

Peaches

Pears

Plums

Orange

Dates

Removed

Sugar apples (chermoya)

Nuts & seeds

Recently added

Hemp seed

Brazil nuts

Previously existing

Walnuts

Raw sesame seeds

Raw sesame "tahini" butter

Removed

Hazelnuts

Raw almonds and almond butter

Pine nuts

Oils

Recently added

Avocado oil

Grapeseed oil

Hempseed oil

Sesame oil

Previously existing

Coconut oil

Olive oil

Spices – seasonings

Recently added

Sweet basil

Habanero

Savory

Previously existing

Basil

Dill

Cloves

Thyme

Bay leaf

Cayenne/african bird pepper

Onion powder

Pure sea salt

Sage

Powdered granulated seaweed

Oregano

Achiote

Tarragon

Removed

Cumin

Coriander

Cilantro

Marjoram

Allspice Parsley

Sugars

Previously existing

Date "sugar

100% pure agave syrup – (from cactus)

Removed

Maple "sugar"

100% pure maple syrup – grade b is recommended

Alkaline grains

Recently added

Fonio

Previously existing

Quinoa

Tef

Kamut

Spelt

Amaranth

Wild rice

Rye

Removed

Black rice

All-natural herbal teas

Recently added

Burdock

Muicle

Cuachalalate

Gordo lobo

Flor de manita

Previously existing

 elderberry

Chamomile

Red raspberry

Ginger

Fennel

Removed

Anise

Lemon grass

Alvaca

Tea leaves

1. Burdock
2. Chamomile
3. Elderberry
4. Fennel
5. Ginger
6. Raspberry
7. Tila

Grains

1. Amaranth
2. Fonio
3. Kamut
4. Quinoa
5. Rye
6. Spelt
7. Teff
8. Wild rice

Spices and Condiments

Mild-flavored spices

1. Basil
2. Bay leaf
3. Cloves

4. Thyme

5. Oregano

6. Dill

7. Savory

8. Sweet basil

9. Tarragon

Spicy flavors

1. Achiote

2. African Bird pepper or cayenne pepper

3. Habanero

4. Sage

5. Onion powder

Salty flavors

1. Sea salt (must be pure and not processed at all)

2. Granulated seaweed (can be consumed in powder form)

3. Kelp, nori, or any other seaweed (they can have a sea taste, which might not be very appealing)

Sweet flavors

1. Agave syrup, which is extracted from cactus (must be pure and not processed at all)

2. Date sugar

Foods to Avoid on the Diet

Foods that are not listed in the nutritional guide are not allowed to be consumed. Some examples of such foods are given below:

1. Any canned product, be it fruits or vegetables, listed in the nutritional guide
2. Seedless fruits like grapes
3. Eggs are not permitted
4. Any type of dairy product is not allowed
5. Fish is not permitted
6. Any type of poultry is not to be eaten
7. Red meat is strictly banned
8. Soy products, which are a replacement for meat, are also banned
9. Processed foods are not allowed
10. Restaurant foods and delivered foods are not to be consumed
11. Hybrid and fortified foods are not permitted
12. Wheat is not permitted
13. White sugar is strictly banned
14. Alcohol is banned
15. Yeast and its products are not allowed
16. Baking powder is not permitted

Some other foods and ingredients have been cut off. You only need to follow the nutritional guide to know what you have to eat.

A Note on Supplements

You need to take Dr. Sebi's supplements daily, alongside your medications, and a daily diet of alkaline food groups. It is mentioned on the website that Dr. Sebi's mixtures/products can release their effects for 14 to 15 days, but there is no scientific data on the matter. Guidelines on nutrients are not present in this diet, so you might have to take extra supplements apart from Dr. Sebi's supplements.

Chapter 5: Strategies of Dr. Sebi's High Blood Pressure Diet

Dr. Sebi discovered many things during his lifetime. He also taught a lot of people many things. During his life, he did many interviews and performed at a lot of speaking engagements where he shared his secrets. Here, we will discuss his top ten diet secrets.

We have to go back to the mother.

Dr. Sebi wrote a paper many years ago called Back to the Mother. In this, he talks about how the land provides for us in a specific manner. He speaks specifically about Africans and how they originally only had the land to live off of. That land provided the foods that they survived with, and that didn't include things like cows, potatoes, beans, yams, lambs, or rice. The lamb came from Arabia and the cow came from Europe. The foods that they ate were electric, and that is what their body needs and that is what kept them healthy. Today, people have strayed from those ways because now they have access to foods from all over the world. Dr. Sebi explained this by saying that "you don't feed gorillas polar bear food." The problems we have are because we have been given the wrong types of foods. This is the main point of his diet. He wants us to go back to the foods that our bodies want us to eat so that it can work properly and to its full capacity.

If you take a look at how other animals eat, you will start to notice something very different. Polar bears feed on seals. Hummingbirds feed on the nectar in flowers. Giraffes eat leaves. Among animals, you have herbivores and carnivores. But when it comes to humans, we don't eat the way our people ate centuries ago when food wasn't as prevalent. That means we aren't giving our bodies what it needs because we can't decide if we need meats or if we need herbs.

Fasting is key to healing your body from disease.

When people hear the word fasting, they instinctively get defensive. When people think fasting, they think starvation, but that isn't what happens when you fast the Dr. Sebi way. Dr. Sebi fasted for 90 days and it helps to cure his diabetes and impotency. During those 90 days, he learned exactly what it was that people needed in order to heal. During this time, he began to drink his urine, lost his eyesight, but continued to do what he was supposed to be doing. Then, four days later his eyesight returned.

This is when he started to have everybody fast that was sick, which included his mother. This helped to cure her diabetes and cleared out her excess mucus in 57 days. Fasting does not mean that you give up food altogether. There are actually many different types of fast, and simply eating only the foods in his nutritional guide will put your body into a state of fasting. You can take things a step further by cutting out most foods except for dates when you are feeling rather weak and drinking bromide plus tea along with plain salads. Fasting is a wonderful thing, and you can experiment with fasting to see what works best for you.

The body works properly through chemical affinity.

During the trial in the late '80s that Dr. Sebi had to face, he asked the judge if it wasn't true that science had proven the body was carbon-based, and that for a carbon-based being to function correctly it needs carbon-based foods. This is what science calls chemical affinity. The body is only able to accept things that it is made of, not something new or alien to it. The foods can provide you with what your body needs are electric foods. The body likes these foods because it makes its chemical makeup.

There is only one disease, and that is excess mucus.

While this is quite possibly the most controversial part of Dr. Sebi's teachings, he has said time and time again that the only disease is too much mucus. When it comes to diseases like diabetes, HIV/AIDS, lupus, and so on, they are created by the body creating too much mucus in a certain area. The body needs mucus, and it contains several mucous membranes that keep things lubricated. When we eat the wrong foods or do things that cause our bodies to become acidic, that mucus starts to grow. The illness that you develop will depend on where all of that mucus begins to grow.

For people with diabetes, the pancreas is where the mucous grows. For something like bronchitis, the mucus is in the lungs. During his trial in the '80s, he asked the judge if she had ever been to an AIDS ward, and she told him yes. Then he asked what the AIDS patients spit up, and she replied with "mucus." That is the basis for his diet is to cleanse the cells of all of this excess mucus to help heal the body from diseases.

Sick people need large doses of iron phosphate.

Dr. Sebi, when asked by potential patients where they should start, he always tells them to start taking iron, which is found in his Bio Ferra product. Iron phosphates are what help the cells to remain healthy once they have been freed of their excess mucus. Modern medicine tends to give people lots of ferrous oxides. Iron is the only magnetic mineral on the planet. Iron pulls all other minerals to it, so when you take iron, you are taking all other minerals as well.

Carbon, hydrogen, and oxygen are the main players in maintaining life.

This may seem extremely obvious because we are taught this in elementary science classes. Everything that the Universe creates is made up of carbon, hydrogen, and oxygen. Those are the main players in making something organic, and these are often missing from things that are created in a lab. These substances do not have starch in them. All substances that are created by Universe, and that are organic, will not contain starch.All of these foods that are naturally present on the Earth, that was made the Universe, are all alkaline foods. These are all-natural. Our blood and body prefer to be fed by these foods because it does not like starch. Starch is only present because it binds things together. Things only have to be bound together if they are not meant to naturally be together.

You have to cleanse and then rebuild the body.

Dr. Sebi's diet works in two parts. First, when you start following his diet you will be cleansing your cells, which he called inter-cellular cleansing. This is what removes toxins and impurities from your body, which will in turn help to heal you from any diseases you are suffering from. Once the cells in your body have been cleansed, it will move into the second part, which rebuilding the body. This means that the body is brought back to its optimal functioning, and most likely to a state that you have never known. The best way for your body to be able to rebuild itself is through the use of iron. If you make sure that your iron level is where it is supposed to be, then you cannot get sick.

Spinach is not a true iron-rich food because it is not alkaline.

As you know already, iron is a very important part of Dr. Sebi's diet. Most everybody will tell you that spinach is a great source of iron, but Dr. Sebi will tell you it is not. Spinach is acidic food. It falls below a 6 on the pH scale because it has a starch base. That means it is not natural. The Universe didn't naturally make this so it is not a good source of iron and will not help your body in any way. On the other hand, moringa has 25 times the amount of iron than spinach does and is not acidic. It also has 14 times the amount of calcium as milk.

The original doctor, Hypocrites, didn't use chemicals, but herbs.

People have fought the notion of Dr. Sebi's diet for years. To them, it doesn't make sense that people would try to heal themselves with diet and herbs since we have doctors. What they don't realize is that the father of modern medicine, Hypocrites, did things very similar to Dr. Sebi. Back when Hypocrites started practicing medicine, they didn't have the chemicals we have now. He didn't give everybody antibiotics whenever they had the sniffles. They didn't have chemotherapy or radiation. All he had to use were things that grew naturally around him. He wouldn't be considered the father of modern medicine if he hadn't been a successful doctor, yet his practice was very different from today. So, if you, or anybody you know, want to shake your head at the teachings of Dr. Sebi, just remember that Hypocrites would support what he is doing.Now you have the ten secrets of Dr. Sebi's diet. While he may have been a completely self-educated man, we knew what he was talking about. Through common sense and personal studies, he created something that has helped many people.

Chapter 6: Approved Products

While food plays the biggest part in the Dr. Sebi diet, there are products that he recommends you take. Various sites sell Dr. Sebi supplements. Some are more expensive than others, but they are all the same things. The goal of the supplements is to provide your body with nutrients that it needs to function properly. Some supplements are specific to men and women as well, so make sure that you pay attention. Most websites will also provide you with grouped products that provide you everything you need for general health or to heal a specific ailment.

Advanced Package

On drsebicellfood.com, they have an advanced package that you can purchase. This advanced package helps provide certain elements to your cells and body to help speed up your healing process. This package helps to engage and revitalize intercellular advancement and it helps to ease the side effects of detoxification. This package contains ten supplements:

- Iron plus

- Green food

- Viento

- Bromide plus capsules

- Bio ferro capsules

- Lupulo

- Focus capsules

- Lymphalin

- Chelation 1

- Chelation 2

All-Inclusive for Women

They also have an all-inclusive package for women. This package is recommended for every woman who wants to follow Dr. Sebi's diet because it helps to cleanse the cellular level of the body by breaking down calcifications, toxins, mucus, and acid. It can then help to restore and rebuild the body, which includes the immune system and blood. This particular package will provide you with the most saturation rate. The higher the saturation rate is, the more effective and faster the cleansing will be. The package has 20 supplements that include:

- Estro

- Endocrine

- Iron plus (2)

- Viento

- Green food

- Bio ferro capsules

- Bromide plus powder

- Bromide plus capsules

- Bio ferro tonic (2)

- Banju (2)

- Lupulo

- Lymphalin

- L.O.V

- Fucus liquid

- Focus capsules

- Chelation 1

- Chelation 2

All-Inclusive for Men

They have an all-inclusive package for men as well. It aims to do the same thing that the female package does, and it contains all of the same supplements except instead of estro you get testo.

Booster Package

If you don't feel like you want to jump all in yet, they have a booster package. The booster package helps to build up the restorative processes in your body. It is customized to help further strengthen your detoxification and intercellular healing. There are seven supplements in this package, which include:

- Green food

- Viento

- Bromide plus capsules

- Bio ferro capsules

- Focus liquid

- Lymphalin

- Chelation 2

Small Cleansing Package

You can also choose from a small cleansing package. This contains Viento, bio Ferro, and chelation 2. This is made to help nourish and cleanse your cellular body. It will help your body get rid of acids, toxins, and mucus that accumulates through your body. It also helps to purify and nourish the blood and helps to bring your body back to a healthier state. This is not considered to be a therapeutic package. If you have certain health problems, you will need to contact their offices to create a therapeutic package that will help your specific concerns.

Support Package

Lastly, they have a support package. This package is meant to introduce the restorative processes to your body. It is made to help provide detoxification and intercellular healing. It contains five supplements, which include:

- Viento

- Bromide plus capsules

- Bio ferro capsules

- Lymphalin

- Chelation 2

Those are just some examples of packages of Dr. Sebi supplements that you can get. You can create your combination of supplements as well. Let's take a moment to go over the individual products that you can choose from.

- Herbal Capsules

VientoViento is working as a revitalize, cleanser, and energizer. It contains chaparral, which is considered to be a powerful antioxidant. Native Americans have used Chaparral for centuries to help treat issues like pain caused by arthritis, snake bites, chickenpox, and respiratory illnesses. Since chaparral has so many antioxidants, it can help with overall wellbeing, weight loss, improve immunity, cleanse the blood, and improve the health of the liver. It has commonly been used to help treat respiratory tract problems and digestive issues like gas and cramps. The herbs found in viento include:

- Hombre grande

- Hierba del Sapo

- Valeriana

- Bladderwrack

- Chaparral

Iron Plus

Iron plus is meant to help purify the entire body. It contains chaparral, which, as we have talked about, is a powerful antioxidant. Iron plus also contains:

- Bugleweed

- Palo guaco

- Hombre grande

- Blue vernvain

- Chaparral

- Elderberry

Green Food

This is a multi-mineral supplement that is made up of herbs from Africa and offers a chlorophyll rich food that nourished the body. It contains ortiga, which is well known as an anti-inflammatory. It can also help with gout, rheumatism, influenza, hemorrhage, cardiovascular system, locomotor system disorders, gastrointestinal tract disorders, urinary tract infections, and kidney disorders. It is also great at helping poor circulation and purifying the blood. Ortiga has also been used to help the symptoms of hay fever. Green food contains:

- Bladderwrack

- Nopal

- Tila

- Nettle

Bromide Plus Powder/Bromide Plus Capsules

This is meant to help your thyroid gland and bones. It is great for people who suffer from dysentery, respiratory issues, pulmonary illnesses, and bad breath. It is a natural diuretic, improves the digestive system, regulates the bowels, and suppresses the appetite. It contains bladderwrack, which is a seaweed that lives in the Baltic Sea, Atlantic Ocean, and the Pacific Ocean. It is one of the sources of iodine. It is full of mannitol, alginic, potassium, bromine, and beta-carotene. It contains bladderwrack and Irish sea moss.

You can also get the bromide plus in capsule form if you would prefer not to drink it as a tea. They both do the same thing for your body and contain the same ingredients. They are simply taken in different ways.

Bio Ferro Tonic/Bio Ferro Capsules

Bio Ferro contains the right ingredients to purify and nourish the blood. It contains a yellow dock root, which is an herb that acts as a digestive bitter to help improve digestion. It is a detoxifier and blood purifier and especially helps the liver. Yellow dock root also helps the digestion of fats and stimulates bile production. It can also help with bowel movements and get rid of waste lingering in the intestinal tract. It will also increase urination. Bio Ferro contains:

- Cocolmeca

- Yellow dock root

- Burdock root

- Chaparral

- Elderberry

The bio ferro capsules work the same way as the tonic. They have slightly different ingredients even though they do the same thing. The capsules contain:

- Yellow dock root

- Nopal

- Nettle

- Burdock root

- Chaparral

Banju

The banjo tonic is made from powerful ingredients to make a tonic that helps to stimulate the central nervous system and brain. It contains:

- Bugleweed

- Valerian root

- Burdock root

- Blue vervain

- Elderberry

Body Care

Uterine Oil and Wash

As you can guess by the name, this is meant for women. This helps to cleanse and restore the flora and fauna of the vagina. The red clover in the wash acts as a blood purifier, improves circulation, and acts as an expectorant. It also contains isoflavones and flavonoids, which help to produce estrogen. Red clover is great at treating conditions that are associated with menopause. The ingredients in the wash include:

- Red clover

- Sage

- Arnica

- Lupulo

Tooth Powder

This is a natural powder that you can use as a toothpaste that will help stop gum disease and tooth decay. It contains Encino and myrrh gum powder.

Testo

It helps to support the male hormonal balance. It also improves your stamina, endurance, and strength. It also helps your prostate health, healthy blood flow to the penis, and improves sexual desire. It contains:

- Irish sea moss

- Capadulla

- Locust bark

- Yohimbi

- Sarsaparilla

Hair Food Oil

This is meant to nourish the scalp and hair. It is gentle on the skin, so it can be used every day. It helps stimulate hair growth. It contains:

- French vanilla

- Coconut oil

- Batana

- Olive oil

Eyewash

This product naturally cleanses and nourishes the eye. It contains the only eyebright, which is commonly used to help treat many different eye diseases. It can also help to reduce the inflammation in the eye caused by conjunctivitis and blepharitis.

Eva Salve

This salve is meant to tone and nourish the skin. The unique combination of ingredients in eva salve provides natural minerals the skin needs like potassium phosphate, fluorine, and calcium, which your skin needs to maintain elasticity. It also contains sage which is a powerful antioxidant that helps to fight off free radical damage. Eva salve contains:

- Manzo

- Eucalyptus

- Sage

- Arnica

- Olive oil

- Lily of the valley

- Nopal

- Shea butter

- Estro

This one is for the ladies and is a natural anti-inflammatory and antioxidant. It contains damiana which has 22 different flavonoids. For centuries, damiana has been used as an aphrodisiac. It can also help to increase and maintain healthy levels of physical and mental stamina. Estro contains:

- Irish sea moss

- Sarsaparilla

- Damiana

- Hydrangea

Herbal Teas

Stomach Relief Tea

This tea contains only cuachalalate, which is an herb used in Central

America that helps provide relief for kidney sickness, gastric ulcers, stomach cancer, and other gastric and stomach pain. This can also help people find relief from kidney and urinary discomfort, minor wounds, and mouth diseases.

Stress Relief Tea

This is simply a chamomile tea which helps to provide a gentle sleeping and relaxation aid. Chamomile works as a mild sedative and can also help to improve a person's mood. It relaxes tense muscles and reduces irritability. It can also help with many stomach troubles, including IBS. It also works as an antioxidant, anti-bacterial, and anti-inflammatory.

Immune Support Tea

This tea provides you with the antioxidant benefits of elderberry. Elderberries are great at reducing the swelling in the mucous membranes. It can also help relieve nasal congestions, and act as an anti-carcinogen and antiviral. It boosts the immune system. Elderberry can also help with any respiratory issue, viral and bacterial infections, flu, colds, coughs, sore throats, improve vision, and lower cholesterol.

Energy Booster Tea

This tea is meant to help boost your energy levels. It can also help to increase your iron levels, which will help to carry more oxygen throughout your body. It contains muicle, which is detoxifying and an antioxidant, and it also acts as a blood purifier.

Cold and Cough Tea

This tea contains gordolobo, which provides you with the relief of mullein flowers that help to ease mucus associated with the flu or cold. Since it helps to reduce phlegm, it will also relieve coughing. It can also help treat intestinal disorders, sore throat, fever, pneumonia, laryngitis, and bronchitis.

Blood Pressure Balance Tea

This tea is made from flor de manita, which helps to regular high or low blood pressure. These flowers have been used for centuries to help heart irregularities and abdominal pain. Regularly consuming this tea could help to lower your cholesterol levels and improve your cardiovascular health.

All of these supplements serve a purpose for your body and helps to improve your overall health. You get the most benefit when you combine the supplements with the Dr. Sebi diet.

Chapter 7: The Doctor Sebi Diet and Weight Loss

Numerous individuals endeavor prevailing fashion diets or those which guarantee snappy outcomes trying to get in shape. These diets may create brings about the present moment, yet after some time, this can be an exceptionally unhealthy approach to get thinner. Also, numerous individuals recover the weight when they go off their exacting diet. At the point when an acid diet is utilized for weight loss and control, it is all the more a way of life change. The outcomes may not occur without any forethought. However, the weight won't be recovered. An alkaline diet is wealthy in nourishments, which are generally low in calories, for example, most vegetables and natural products. A significant number of the nourishments that are high in fat and calories are likewise acidifying, so when these nourishments are expelled from the diet, a characteristic and healthy weight loss will happen. These nourishments incorporate red meat, greasy food sources, and high-fat dairy items, for example, whole milk and cheddar, sugar, pop, and liquor. When you quit eating these nourishments, your body will be a lot healthier, less acid, and you'll additionally get more fit all the while. Since the diet is healthy, you can stay with it long haul. Numerous individuals who start an alkaline diet exclusively to get in shape find countless different advantages. An expanded energy level, protection from an ailment, and a general improvement in health and prosperity are among the numerous benefits you can understand on an alkaline diet.

Alkaline Diet for Health and Weight Loss

There are a ton of insane diets available that guarantee to assist you with shedding pounds. Shockingly, on the off chance that you take a gander at the healthy benefit of a portion of these diets, they are regularly seriously deficient. If you have to get thinner, you ought to do it while eating food that is useful for your body, with the goal that you will get healthier rather than merely more slender. An alkaline diet is a healthy way to deal with weight loss that will keep you stimulated, healthy, and inspired to drop the pounds.

An alkaline diet is not the same as different diets since it centers mostly around the impact that nourishments have on the acidity or the alkalinity of the body. At the point when nourishments are processed and used by the body, they produce what is usually alluded to as an "alkaline debris" or "acid debris." The first pH of the nourishment doesn't factor into this decisive impact inside the body. The absolute most acidic nourishments, for example, organic citrus products, really produce an alkaline effect when eaten. At the point when increasingly alkaline nourishments are eaten instead of acid nourishments, the pH of the body can be acclimated to an ideal degree of roughly 7.3. While this isn't incredibly alkaline, it is sufficient to receive numerous healthful rewards.

Alkaline Diet Can Save Your Life

Most vegetables and organic products contain a higher measure of essential shaping components than different nourishments. The more noteworthy the ratio of green nourishments devoured in the diet, the more prominent the health benefits accomplished. These plant nourishments are purifying and alkalizing to the body, while the refined and handled nourishments can increment unhealthy degrees of acidity and poisons. Be that as it may, know that an excess of alkaline can likewise hurt you. You should have the best possible information on adjusting alkaline and acidic nourishments in your diet. After ingestion, alkaline nourishment and water are very quickly killed by hydrochloric acid present in the stomach. The harmony among alkaline and acidic nourishments must be kept up all together for your organs to perform well.

A healthy and adjusted diet is more alkaline than acid. Given your blood classification, the menu ought to be comprised of 60 to 80% alkaline nourishments and 20 to 40% acidic food sources. Typically, the A and AB blood classifications require the most alkaline diet, while the O and B blood classifications require creature items increasingly in their diet. In any case, remember, in case you're in torment, you're acidic. Progressing to an alkaline diet requires a move in one's mentality about nourishment. It is useful to investigate new tastes and surfaces while rolling out little improvements and improving old propensities.

The Perks of the Alkaline Diet Program

Society today is assaulted by such a significant number of various diet programs that it very well may be overpowering. A few diets place limitations on what nourishments can be eaten due to what's in them, while others are progressively indulgent with nourishment determination, however stringent on when you can eat. The reason for diets differs too, and some are intended to get more fit and others are for improving health. The alkaline diet can be grouped into the last mentioned, as it comprises of expending healthy nourishments yet can at the previous outcome in weight loss too.

The pH level of the human body should be around 7.35, which is somewhat alkaline and implies that alkaline is required by the body. Trackers and gatherers, a longtime prior, experienced no difficulty addressing this need as the vast majority of the nourishments they are were wealthy in alkaline, for example, vegetables, nuts, and seeds.

These days notwithstanding, the cutting-edge diet isn't exceptionally alkaline, comprising mainly of handled nourishments and creature protein. At the point when these nourishments and different things, for example, espresso, beans, and fish, are expended, they discharge acids that happen to debilitate our bones.

The alkaline diet is engaging because it advances quality during the bones and joints. Acid debilitates the bones, so expending a diet high in alkaline will balance the impacts that acids have on our bodies. That is the reason this diet contains nourishments, for example, natural products, seeds, nuts, green tea, tomatoes, etc. because they have low degrees of acid. However, more grounded joints and bones aren't the main advantages of the alkaline diet.

Extra advantages of the alkaline diet incorporate expanded energy levels and hindering an abundance of mucous generation. It can likewise enable the individuals to experience the ill effects of this season's flu virus, colds, and nasal clog as often as possible. Also, the individuals who have different indications, for example, polycystic ovaries, ovarian pimples, and kindhearted bosom growths, can improve by changing to an alkaline-based diet. At last, it can decrease sentiments of crabbiness, uneasiness, and tension.

Chapter 8: How to Naturally Reverse Your Diabetes: Dr. Sebi Natural Food Guide to End Diabetes

Although it is quite difficult to plan a diabetes food as it does not necessarily need to have a taste or to be boring, with just a little direction, a diet plan that is both nutritional and appetizing can be conjured up.

Diet Planning

A dietetic plan should make sure that all the carbohydrates are taken each diet every day is well spread out so as not to engulf the body system. This is vital as it assists in making sure that the blood sugar levels are kept in control. Therefore, there is a requirement to stay on the pathway of what is being eaten.

The number of carbs eaten can also be controlled while making use of insulin and performing exercise. The majority of the diabetic patent have to be worried about the sodium content of the foods they eat, as it is possible that it can play a negative part in the high blood pressure, which is presently in the majority of diabetic patients.

Those with an extra medical condition of hypertension would be conscious of taking in sodium. For diabetic patients with high levels of lipids while taking in saturated fats, cholesterol, and trans-fat would be watched.

While trying to create a meal plan for a diabetic patient, some basic points should be taken notice of. These might add to ensuring that the calories which are taking in are kept to about 10% to 20% coming from a protein source.

Meats, which include beef and chicken, should be thought about over other options. About 25% to 30% of the calories should emerge from fats. However, foods that have saturated and trans fats should either be eaten in bits or totally shun. About 50% to 60% of calories should emerge from carbohydrates. Taking in plenty of oranges and green vegetables will assist you to sustain the balance, they may include the likes of broccoli or carrots. Taking in sweet potatoes or brown rice is preferable rather than regular potatoes and white rice because it is more advisable to eat as it serves as a nutritional benefit.

Dr. Sebi Herbal Supplements for Type 2 Diabetes

This is a disease that builds because of the issue associated with the hormone insulin, which is produced by the pancreas. In cases where this process is interrupted due to irregularity, there is not enough control of the glucose in the blood and the amount that is taken into the cell. However, there are a few of the medical and home remedies that can be taken a look at to control this abnormality within the body.

Natural Sugar Control

Outlined below are a few recommendations of home remedies that should be taken a look at when you want to reduce the problems of diabetic patients:

- Taking Alpha lipoid acid assists in managing the sugar level in the blood, and it is seen as one of the best multipurpose antioxidants.

- Taking 400mcg a day. Chromium picolinate helps insulin to keep the sugar levels in the body low. The Chromium picolinate keeps the blood sugar level when you take the right insulin.

- Taking garlic is another essential method of assisting the circulation and control of sugar levels. It comes in suitable capsules for easy and stress-free consumption.

- 500mg of L-glutamine and taurine each day will assist in bringing down the sugar cravings and also help to release the insulin the right way. It is useful for people who have problems managing their intake of sweet food items.

- Huckleberry is the best option for improving the production of insulin in the body when it is taken with the right prescription. It is a natural remedy that is recommended for consumption.

- A mixture of tea and kidney beans, navy beans, white beans, lima beans, and northern beans does assist in eliminating the toxin from the pancreas.

There are more natural remedies that are used in managing blood sugar levels in diabetic patients. Meanwhile, the listed remedies should be consumed with either medical authorization or advice from some experts who have a deep understanding of the diabetic disease.

Type 2 diabetes affects over 30 million Americans – and the diabetes epidemic shows no sign of getting eradicated. When a patient is suffering from type 2 diabetes, it requires the sugar level to be controlled. When diet and exercise fail to control the blood sugar level, medications like metformin becomes an alternative. But with the breakthrough Dr. Sebi gave in his research for alternative medicines that help cure diabetes, we now have a huge list of herbal medicines that can not only control the blood sugar level but has the potentials to cure it totally.

The research of these herbs has been proven to work in treating type 2 diabetes. According to Dr. Sebi, a combination of electric food is what is needed to keep the body's alkalinity at the level it needs to repel mucus.

Root Vegetables and Fruits for Diabetics

Because of the several health problems that can happen in the body of a diabetic, it is necessary to be careful with the diet plan taken every day.

Fruits and Veggies

Any consumption of food needs to be done with some level of sensitivity to make sure it is the best for the diabetics. Every diabetic patient needs to make sure they follow the balanced diet which is rich in minerals and vitamins. Also, the foods which have protein, fats, and carbs should be at an acceptable level.

Root vegetables and fruits have been taken as a huge source of minerals and vitamins and fiber which is vital in reducing the chances of heart attack and stroke occurring chances. These root vegetables and fruits generally assist in making up for any side effects the distressed blood sugar level causes. These side effects are expected to lead to heart attacks and blindness if not managed effectively by the regulating ingredients of minerals and vitamins gotten from the root vegetables and fruits.

It should be taken into notice that eating root vegetables and fruits is a mixture of other food items that are seen as the best for diabetic patient consumption rather than eating them without taking in snacks. It is so because when these root vegetables are eaten together with other foods, the chemical reactions will let all the vitamins and the minerals to be easily absorbed in the body system and this will lead to a controlled blood sugar level.

However, when it is taken in as a standalone item like snacks, the blood sugar levels are likely to be increased as the absorption levels will be twisted and lower than optimum. The most vital point to take notice of is to make sure that any food you eat should be done in a mixture that lets the absorption levels to be the best for the patient with diabetics to take in.

Chapter 9: Tips for successfully follow the Dr Sebi diet

Often, stretching for the additional mile, you get to the areas you had only dreamed about. Going well on an alkaline diet will be the battle that ultimately contributes to a balanced lifestyle. An alkaline diet is an assumption that certain products, such as berries, vegetables, roots, and legumes, leave an alkaline residue or ash behind in the body. The body is strengthened by the key ingredients of rock, such as calcium, magnesium, titanium, zinc, and copper. The avoidance of asthma, malnutrition, exhaustion, and even cancer is an alkaline diet. Conscious about doing something like that? Here are ten strategies to adopt the alkaline diet effectively.

Drink water

Water is probably our body's most important (after oxygen) resource. Hydration in the body is very important as the water content determines the body's chemistry. Drink between 8-10 glasses of water to keep the body well hydrated (filtered to cleaned).

Avoid acidic drinks like Tea, coffee, or soda

Our body also attempts to regulate acid and alkaline content. There is no need to blink in carbonated drinks as the body refuses carbon dioxide as waste!

Breathe

Oxygen is the explanation that our body works, and if you provide the body with adequate oxygen, it should perform better. Sit back and enjoy two to five minutes of slow breaths. Nothing is easier than you can perform Yoga.

Avoid food with preservatives and food colors

Our body has not been programmed to absorb such substances, and the body then absorbs them or retains them as fat, and they do not damage the liver. Chemicals create acids, such that the body neutralizes them either by generating cholesterols or blanching iron from the RBCs (leading to anemia) or by extracting calcium from bones (osteoporosis).

Avoid artificial Sweeteners

These sweeteners, which tend to be high in low fat, are potentially detrimental to the body. In addition, Saccharin, a primary ingredient in sweeteners, triggers cancer. Keep away from these things, therefore. Go for less healthy food, still a decent one.

Exercise

The alkaline and the acidic element will also be matched. This is not just a question of consuming alkaline milk. A little acid (because of muscles) often regulates natural bodywork.

Satiate your urges for a snack by eating vegetables, or soaked nuts

Whenever we are thirsty, we still consume a little fast food. Establish a tradition of consuming fresh vegetables or almonds, even walnuts.

Eat the right mix of food

The fats and proteins of carbohydrates need a specific atmosphere when digested. And don't eat it all at once. Evaluate the nutritional composition and balance it accurately to create the best combination of all the nutrients you consume.

Sleep well, remain calm and composed even when under stress

Seek to escape the pain. Our mind regulates the digestive system, and only when in a relaxed, focused condition can you realize it functions properly. Relax, then, and remain safe!

Have a better understanding of what an alkaline diet is.

It is really interesting to learn what the alkaline diet entails. We should remember that an Alkaline diet mainly comprises fresh fruits and vegetables, which, once metabolized in our bodies, produce alkaline residues. Meat, including beef, pork, and other processed ingredients, does not come from alkaline eating items and must also be consumed in minimal amounts.

Plan for your meals ahead of time.

Preliminary preparation of the meals is a healthy way to thoroughly value and sustain successful eating habits. It is essential that you mention the foods you need to prioritize. Although it will take some time while you do so, it will be beneficial as you have enough opportunity to reflect and write down things that can lead you to a healthy lifestyle and to consume better.

Eat plenty of vegetables and fruits.

Because alkaline foods are mainly fruits and vegetables, more can be consumed. Such foods have negatively charged components that neutralize the acids that are charged positively when taken in by our bodies. The muscle, on the other side, retains a pH equilibrium. There are also some acidic fruit and vegetables that are not recommended to consume in large quantities.

Know the importance of pH balance.

If we recognize the value of maintaining a pH balance, we should be careful with the kinds of food we eat. The fluids in our body have to retain a healthy pH degree such that our cells will continue to work properly. It does not mean, however, that we finally should not eat acid foods. To get a healthy body state, 75%–80% of alkaline, and 20%–25% of acid products must be consumed.

Improving your life doesn't require much time, but you will create major improvements in your lifestyle with the right awareness. We just need a healthy eating routine with alkaline diet plans. Nobody wants a sedentary life, so now we have to move.

Chapter 10: Soups Recipes

Tangy Lentil Soup

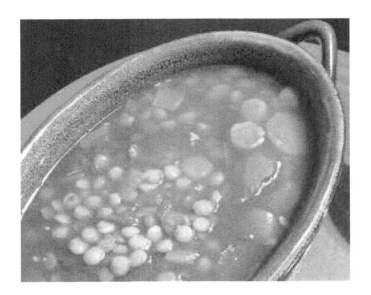

Preparation Time: 5 minutes

Cooking Time: 15 minutes

Serves: 4

Ingredients:

2 cups picked over and rinsed red lentils

1 chopped serrano Chile pepper

1 large chopped and roughly to mato

1-1/2 inch peeled and grated piece ginger

3 finely chopped cloves chive

1/4 tsp. ground turmeric

Sea salt

Topping

1/4 cup coconut yogurt

Instructions:

In a pot add the lentils with enough water to cover the lentils.

Boil the lentils then reduce the heat.

Cook for about 10 minutes on low heat to simmer.

Add the remaining ingredients then stir.

Cook until lentils become soft and properly mixed.

Garnish a dollop of coconut yogurt.

Serve.

Turnip Green Soup

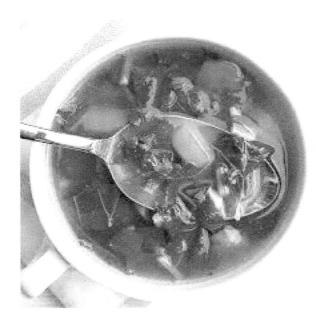

Preparation Time: 5 minutes

Cooking Time: 22 minutes

Serves: 2

Ingredients:

2 tbsps. coconut oil

1 large chopped onion

3 minced cloves chive

2-in piece peeled and minced ginger

3 cups bone broth

1 medium cubed white turnip

1 large chopped head radish

1 bunch chopped kale

1 seville orange, 1/2 zested and juice reserved

1/2 tsp. sea salt

1 bunch cilantro

Instructions:

In a skillet, add oil then heat it.

Add in the onions as you stir.

Sauté for about 7 minutes then add chive and ginger.

Cook for about 1 minute.

Add in the turnip, broth, and radish then stir.

Bring the soup to boil then reduce the heat to allow it to simmer.

Cook for an extra 15 minutes then turn off the heat.

Pour in the remaining ingredients.

Using a handheld blender, pour the mixture.

Garnish with cilantro.

Serve warm.

Lentil Kale Soup

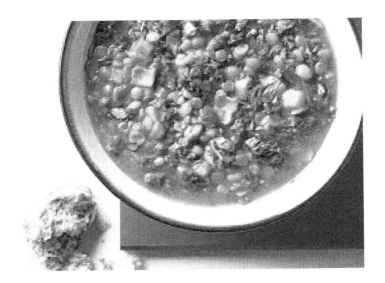

Preparation Time: 5 minutes

Cooking Time: 15 minutes

 Serves: 4

Ingredients:

1/2 Onion

2 Zucchinis

1 rib Celery

1 stalk Chive

1 cup diced tomatoes

1 tsp. dried vegetable broth powder

1 tsp. Sazon seasoning

1 cup red lentils

1 tbsp. Seville orange juice

3 cups alkaline water

1 bunch kale

Instructions:

In a greased pan, pour in all the vegetables.

Sauté for about 5 minutes then add the tomatoes, broth, and Sazon seasoning.

Mix properly then stir in the red lentils together with water.

Cook until the lentils become soft and tender.

Add the kale then cook for about 2 minutes.

Serve warm with the seville orange juice.

Chive Celery Soup

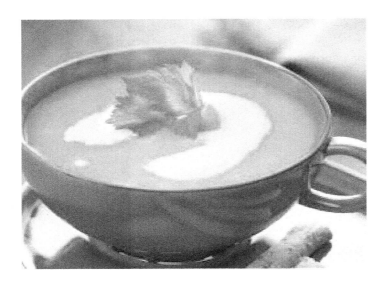

Preparation Time: 15 minutes

Cooking Time: 1 hr. 10 minutes

Serves: 4

Ingredients:

2 peeled and roughly chopped zucchinis

1 roughly chopped onion

2 tsps. sea salt

2 bay leaves

9 cups water

2 cleaned and roughly chopped Celery stalks

5 smashed chive stalks

1 peeled and roughly chopped parsnip

2 chopped celery stalks,

Instructions:

Spray a little cooking spray to the bottom of a stockpot.

Place the stockpot over moderate heat then sauté the onions for 5 about minutes as you stir constantly.

Add the chive, parsnip, celery, and zucchinis to the stockpot.

Sauté for 3 minutes.

Add the bay leaves, salt, and water to stockpot then allow it to simmer for 1 hour.

Remove the stockpot from heat then cool slightly.

Strain out the vegetables, leaving the broth.

When it is ready, serve the soup then add some of the vegetables back into the soup.

Serve.

Pumpkin Squash Soup

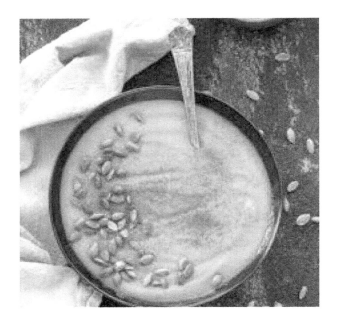

Preparation Time: 5 minutes

Cooking Time: 15 minutes

Serves: 4

Ingredients:

Cayenne pepper, pinch

Sea salt, pinch

Grapeseed oil, 1 tbsp

Vegetable broth, 2.25 c

Basil leaves, .5 c

Chopped fresh ginger, small piece

Diced onion, 1

Coconut cream, 1 c

Butternut squash, peeled and cubed, 4 c

Instructions:

Place large skillet on medium heat. Put grapeseed oil in skillet and warm. Place the onion into the warmed skillet with the ginger and cook until it has softened.

Add butternut squash into the skillet and continue to cook for about ten minutes. Stirring every now and then until squash begins to soften and turn slightly brown.

Add vegetable broth and season with cayenne and salt. Allow to boil and turn heat down. Let simmer about ten minutes until squash is extremely soft.

Gently pour soup into a blender and add the cream. Place lid back onto the blender. Since the liquid is hot, you will need to hold the lid down by using a kitchen towel. Turn the blender on until it becomes smooth.

Ladle into bowls and garnish with basil leaves.

Cauliflower Curry Soup

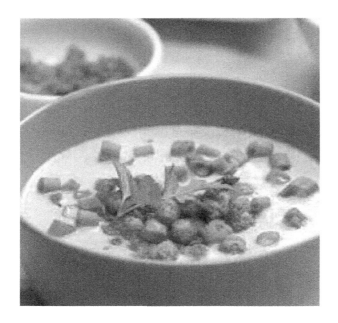

Preparation Time: 10 minutes

 Cooking Time: 45 minutes

Serves: 4

Ingredients:

1 chopped large head of cauliflower

4 tbsps. divided coconut oil

1 diced medium yellow onion

3 tbsps. Thai red curry paste

1/2 tsp. Seville orange zest

1/2 cup unoaked white wine

1-1/2 cups vegetable stock

14 oz. light coconut milk

3 tsps. rice vinegar

Iodine free Celtic sea salt

Freshly ground black pepper

1 tbsp. chopped fresh basil

Nuts

Instructions:

Adjust the temperature of your oven to 400ºF.

In a bowl, mix the cauliflower with coconut oil.

Pour it on a large baking sheet as you spread it.

Bake for 30 minutes.

In a Dutch oven, melt 1 tbsp. coconut oil.

Add onion with a dash of salt to sauté for 3 minutes.

Add in the curry paste and seville orange zest then stir.

Properly mix them then add wine.

Cook until it is completely absorbed

Add the vegetable stock, coconut milk, and the roasted cauliflower.

Cook for 10 minutes on low heat to simmer.

Pour the soup using a handheld blender after cooling it for about 5 minutes.

Add salt and pepper to season.

Garnish the meal with the nuts and basil.

Serve warm.

Zucchini Turnip Soup

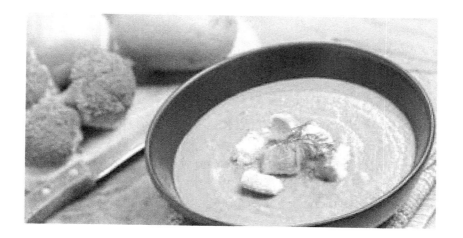

Preparation Time: 10 minutes

Cooking Time: 30 minutes

Serves: 4

Ingredients:

1 tbsp. coconut oil

2 cups chopped yellow onion

2 minced cloves chive

1 tbsp. minced fresh ginger

2 tbsps. red curry paste

4 cups low-sodium vegetable broth

3 cups peeled and diced zucchinis

3 cups peeled and diced turnips

Iodine free Celtic sea salt

Freshly ground black pepper

1/4 tsp. cayenne pepper

Instructions:

Sauté the onion, ginger, and chive in a greased pan for about 6 minutes.

Add in the curry paste then stir and broth.

Mix properly then add the turnips, salt, and zucchinis

Boil the soup on high heat.

Cover the pot.

Cook for about 20 minutes.

Blend this soup in a blender in batches until it becomes smooth.

Add salt and pepper to season.

Serve warm.

Soursop Ginger Soup

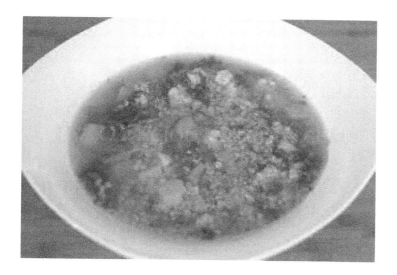

Preparation Time: 5 minutes

Cooking Time: 15 minutes

Serves: 4

Ingredients:

Cayenne, .25 tsp.

Minced ginger, 1 tbsp

Quinoa, 1 c

Diced red pepper, 1 c

Oregano, 1 tbsp

Diced green peppers, 1 c

Basil, 1 tbsp

Diced onions, 1 c

Sea salt, 4 tsp.

Cubed summer squash, 1 c

Onion powder, 3 tbsp

Cubed zucchini, 1 c

Cubed chayote squash, 2 c

Chopped kale, 2 c

Springwater, 1 gallon

Soursop leaves, 4 to 6

Instructions:

Rinse the soursop and rip then in half. Add them to a pot with the water. Boil the leaves for about 15 to 20 minutes.

Take the leaves out.

Add in all of the other ingredients. Add in another eight cups of water.

Mix the ingredients together. Place the lid on and cook it for 30 to 45 minutes.

Roasted Vegetable and Coconut Milk Soup

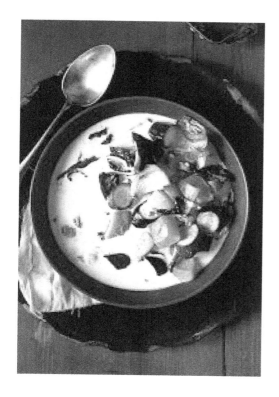

Preparation Time: 5 minutes

Cooking Time: 15 minutes

 Serves: 4

Ingredients:

Cayenne pepper, to taste

Sea salt, to taste

Grapeseed oil, 1 tbsp plus more for vegetables

Coconut milk, 1 c

Grated ginger, 1 tbsp

Diced onion, 1 small

Vegetable of choice, 2 c chopped

Instructions:

Warm your oven to 350. Place your chopped vegetables onto a baking dish. Drizzle with grapeseed oil and toss to coat. Season with pepper and salt. Toss again. Place in the oven and cook 40 minutes.

While vegetables are roasting, cook the sauce. Add grapeseed oil to a skillet and warm. Add onion and let it cook for some time until it gets softened. Add ginger and cook until fragrant.

Now you need to add the coconut milk and let it come to a boil. Lessen the heat and let it continue to simmer about 30 minutes until reduced to the way you want it.

When veggies are done, carefully remove from oven.

Pour milk mixture into two bowls. Divide the vegetables evenly into the bowl. Add more seasonings if desired.

You can mash a few vegetables if you would like to.

Chapter 11: Salads Recipes

Headache Salad

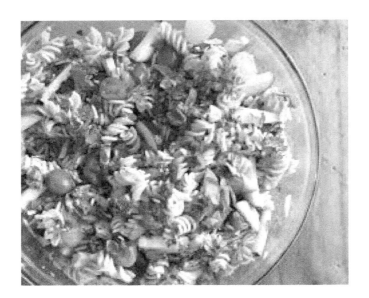

Preparation Time: 10 minutes

Cooking Time: 0 minutes

Serves: 2

Ingredients:

Cayenne pepper, to taste

Salt, to taste

Olive oil, 2 tbsp

Key lime juice, 1 tbsp

Watercress, 2 c

Cucumber, seeded, .5

Instructions:

Place the cucumber and watercress onto a serving plate.

Put the juice and olive oil into a small bowl and whisk until well combined.

Pour over watercress and cucumber. Sprinkle with pepper and salt. Enjoy.

Strawberry Dandelion Salad

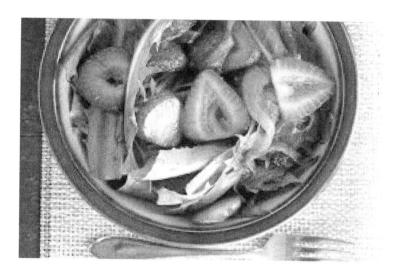

Preparation Time: 10 minutes

Cooking Time: 0 minutes

Serves: 2

Ingredients:

Sea salt, to taste

Dandelion greens, 4 c

Key lime juice, 2 tbsp

Sliced strawberries, 10

Sliced red onion, 1 medium

Grapeseed oil, 2 tbsp

Instructions:

Place a nonstick skillet on top of the stove and warm. Add the onions and a pinch of salt. Cook while stirring until onions are slightly brown and soft.

Place one teaspoon of the lime juice into a small bowl, add in the strawberries and toss to coat.

Wash the dandelion greens and dry them with paper towels. If you prefer, you can tear or cut the greens into smaller pieces.

Once the onions are almost cooked through, add the rest of the lime juice to the onions and cook for about two minutes until onions are coated. Take off heat.

Place the strawberries, onions, and greens in a salad bowl along with all the juices. Sprinkle on some sea salt. Enjoy.

Grilled Romaine Salad

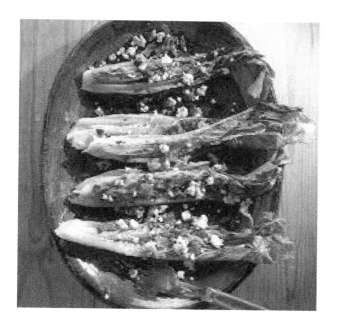

Preparation Time: 10 minutes

Cooking Time: 0 minutes

Serves: 2

Ingredients:

Agave syrup, 1 tbsp

Olive oil, 4 tbsp

Sea salt, to taste

Onion powder, to taste

Key lime juice, 1 tbsp

Cayenne pepper, to taste

Finely chopped red onion, 1 tbsp

Chopped basil, 1 tbsp

Romaine lettuce, 4 small heads, rinsed

Instructions:

Cut each Romaine head in half. Place each half into a nonstick skillet cut side down. You don't need to add oil. Lettuce needs to be browned on each side. Check for doneness by lifting the lettuce up. Once all the lettuce has been browned, take off heat and let it cool on a platter.

To make the dressing: place the basil, lime juice, agave syrup, and olive oil into a small bowl. Whisk to combine. Add cayenne pepper, onion powder, and salt. Whisk again until well combined.

Place the grilled lettuce onto a serving platter and drizzle on the dressing.

Avocado Basil Pasta Salad

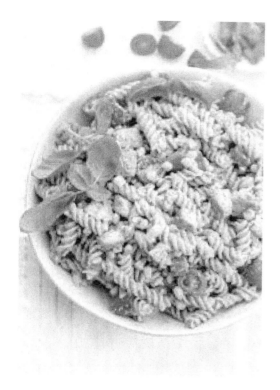

Preparation Time: 15 minutes

Cooking Time: 0 minutes

Serves: 2

Ingredients:

Cooked spelt pasta, 4 c

Olive oil, .25 c

Agave syrup, 1 tsp.

Key lime juice, 1 tbsp

Halved cherry tomatoes, 1 pint

Chopped basil, 1 c

Chopped avocado, 1

Instructions:

Put the cooked pasta into a large bowl.

Add in the tomatoes, basil, and avocado. Toss to combine.

Put the salt, agave syrup, lime juice, and oil into a bowl. You are going to need to whisk everything vigorously in order to get everything combined.

Pour dressing on top of the pasta mixture. Now toss everything together to coat the pasta with the dressing.

Quinoa and Zucchini Salad

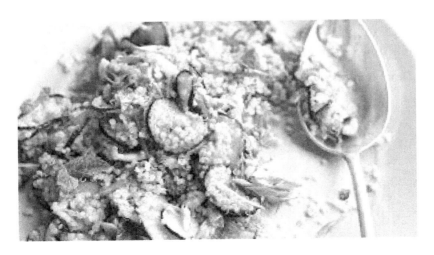

Preparation Time: 15 minutes

Cooking Time: 0 minutes

Serves: 2

Ingredients:

Finely chopped spring onions, 2

Juice of one Key lime

Olive oil, 3 tbsp

Chickpeas, 1 can drained and rinsed

Oregano, 1 tsp.

Grapeseed oil, 2 tbsp

Quinoa, .5 c

Onion powder, 1 tsp.

Sliced zucchini, 2 large

Instructions:

Place the quinoa into a pot and pour in one cup of water. Allow to boil and then turn heat down and simmer until all water is absorbed about ten minutes. Cover with lid and set to the side.

Add grapeseed oil into a larger skillet and let it warm up. Put the zucchini into the pot and let the zucchini cook while you stir until they are tender but still bright green. Place into a bowl and season to taste. Put the skillet back onto the stove. Add the oregano cook while stirring until fragrant. Add this oil to the zucchini.

Add the spring onions, lime juice, olive oil, onion powder, quinoa, and chickpeas to zucchini and toss well.

Cherry Tomato & Kale Salad

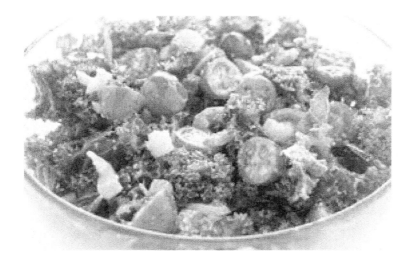

Preparation Time: 10 minutes

Cooking Time: 0 minutes

Serves: 2

Ingredients:

2 tbsps. Ranch dressing

2 cups organic baby tomatoes

1 bunch kale, stemmed, leaves washed and chopped

Instructions:

Mix all the ingredients in a bowl.

Divide the salad equally in two servings dishes.

Serve.

Radish Noodle Salad

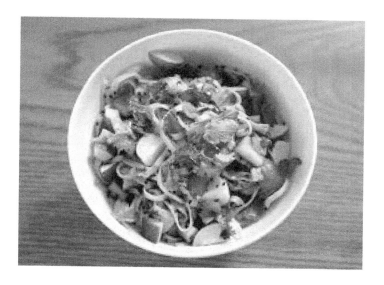

Preparation Time: 10 minutes

Cooking Time: 0 minutes

Serves: 4

Ingredients:

2 cups cooked radish florets

1 roasted spaghetti squash

1 chopped scallion

1 tbsp. sesame oil

1 bell seeded pepper, cut into strips

2 tbsps. toasted sesame seeds

1 tsp. sea salt

1 tsp. red pepper flakes

Instructions:

Start by preparing the spaghetti squash by removing the cooked squash with a fork into a bowl.

Add the radish, red bell pepper, and scallion to the bowl with the squash.

In a small bowl, mix the red pepper flakes, salt, and sesame oil.

Drizzle the mixture to top the vegetables. Toss gently to combine them.

Add the sesame seeds to garnish.

Serve.

Caprese Salad

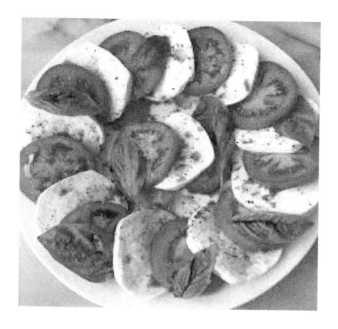

Preparation Time: 5 minutes

Cooking Time: 0 minutes

Serves: 2

Ingredients:

1 sliced avocado

2 sliced large tomatoes

1 bunch basil leaves

1 tsp. sea salt

1 cup cubed jackfruit

Instructions:

In a bowl toss all the salad ingredients to mix.

Add the sea salt to season.

Serve.

Avocado Power Salad

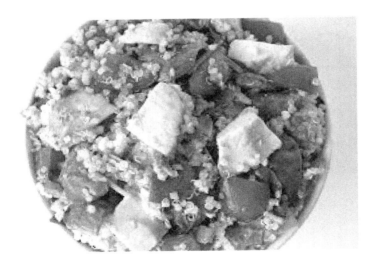

Preparation Time: 10 minutes

Cooking Time: 0 minutes

Serves: 2

Ingredients:

1 cubed avocado

1 cup cooled cooked quinoa

1 tbsp. freshly squeezed seville orange juice

1 tsp. sea salt

1 tbsp. onion powder

1 tbsp. onion powder

1/4 cup chopped cilantro

1 cup peeled and diced cucumber

1 cup halved cherry tomatoes

5oz. fresh and roughly chopped kale

Instructions:

Mix all the ingredients.

Place the mixture in the fridge to chill for about 15 minutes

Serve.

Summer Lettuce Salad

Preparation Time: 5 minutes

Cooking Time: 0 minutes

Serves: 4

Ingredients:

2 cups halved cherry tomatoes

4 cups romaine lettuce or iceberg

1 peeled and sliced cucumber

2 thinly sliced radishes

1 sliced scallion

1/2 cup shredded zucchini

14 oz. can drained whole green beans

Instructions:

Add all of the salad ingredients in a large bowl then toss with 2 tbsps. of the dressing.

Serve.

Citrus Watercress Salad

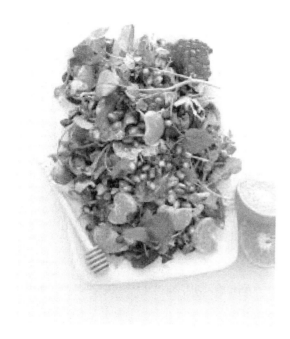

Preparation Time: 10 minutes

Cooking Time: 0 minutes

Serves: 2

Ingredients:

Cayenne pepper, to taste

Salt, dash

Olive oil, 2 tbsp

Juice of one key lime

Agave syrup, 2 tsp.

Thinly sliced red onion, 2

Zest of one Seville orange

Segments of Seville orange

Watercress, 4 c

Avocado, 1

Instructions:

Take two plates and divide out the orange segments, sliced onions, sliced avocados, and watercress evenly.

In a small bowl, place the cayenne pepper, salt, agave syrup, olive oil, and lime juice. Whisk until well combined.

Pour over salad once you are ready to serve.

Chapter 12: Main Dishes Recipes

Irish Sea Moss Alkaline Electric Recipe

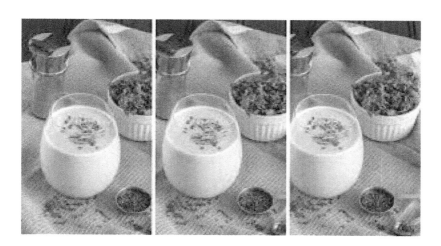

Preparation Time: 10 minutes

Cooking Time: 30 minutes

Serves: 3

Ingredients

2 oz of irish sea moss

2 cupsof clean water

Instructions

Start with 2 oz. of your wild sea moss to make an Irish sea moss gel.

Rinse, then soak in spring water for 24 hours. The sea moss will double in size.

Rinse again and chop into bits to make it easier for your blender.

Add the already soaked sea moss and 2 cups of water to your blend.

You can put it in a jar and refrigerate for several weeks if you wish.

Lasagna

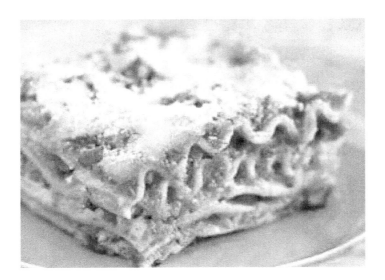

Preparation Time: 10 minutes

Cooking Time: 20 minutes

Serves: 3

Ingredients:

Spelt lasagna sheets

Mushrooms

Zucchini

Tomato Sauce:

Basil, 2 tsp.

Cayenne pepper, .5 tsp.

Onion powder, 1 tbsp

Agave, 1 tbsp

Sea salt, 2 tsp.

Plum tomatoes, 12

Oregano, 2 tsp.

"Meat":

Fennel powder, 1 tsp.

Sea salt, 1 tbsp

Diced red, yellow, and green bell peppers, 1 c

Basil, 2 tsp.

Chopped onions, 1 c

Oregano, 2 tsp.

Cooked garbanzo beans, 1 c

Onion powder, 2 tbsp

Cooked spelt berries, 2 c

Cheese:

Basil, 1 tsp.

Hemp seeds, 1 tbsp

Onion powder, 1 tbsp

Springwater, 1 c

Oregano, 1 tsp.

Soaked brazil nuts, 2 c

Sea salt, 1 tsp.

Instructions:

Start by fixing the tomato sauce. Add all of the tomato sauce ingredients to your blender and mix them together until they form a sauce. Pour this into a pot and allow the sauce to begin boiling. Lower the heat down a bit and let it continue to simmer, stirring occasionally, for at least two hours, or until it has thickened up.

As this cook, you can get the "meat" mixture together. Add the seasonings, garbanzo beans, and spelt to a food processor and mix it all together until it becomes well blended.

Add a skillet to high heat with some grapeseed oil. Mix in the garbanzo bean mixture and let everything cook for ten to 12 minutes. Everything needs to be browning up.

Now place all of the cheese mixture ingredients to your blender and mix them all together until they are well combined. If it appears too thick, add in an extra quarter cup of water slowly until it reaches the consistency you are looking for.

Reserve a cup of the tomato sauce. Add the rest of the sauce to the "meat" mixture and stir everything together. Slice up some zucchini and mushrooms.

Get a glass baking dish and add a bit of the tomato sauce to the bottom to make sure that the pasta doesn't stick to it. Lay down some pasta and top it with zucchini, "meat" mixture, cheese, and then mushrooms. Repeat this process until your lasagna has four layers. Your final layer of lasagna will be covered with the "meat" mixture and then the cheese. Pour the reserved tomato sauce around the lasagna.

Put the lasagna into the preheated oven and let it bake for 35 to 45 minutes at 350. Before you slice the lasagna, let it sit for no less than 15 minutes.

Kale and Brazil Nut Pesto with Butternut Squash

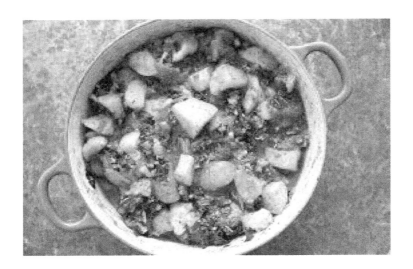

Preparation Time: 10 minutes

Cooking Time: 30 minutes

Serves: 3

Ingredients:

Squash:

Sea salt

Dried sage, 1 tbsp

Grapeseed oil, 1 tbsp

Cubed butternut squash, 1.5 c

Pesto:

Onion powder, 2 tsp.

Chopped Brazil nuts, 2 tbsp

Olive oil, 4 tbsp

Juice of 2 limes

Parsley, 1 tbsp

Kale, 2 c – washed and stem removed

Cooked quinoa, 2.5 c – to serve

Instructions:

To start, get your oven to 400. Add the butternut squash to a bowl and drizzle in the oil. Add in the seasonings and toss everything to squash well. Pour the squash onto a baking sheet and allow it to bake for at least 30 minutes. Once it can be pierced easily with a fork, it is finished.

As the squash is cooking, add the kale, parsley, lime juice, olive oil, brazil nuts, and onion powder to your food processor. Turn the processor on and allow everything to mix together until it all comes together. The pesto may appear dry, but that's okay. This process may be loud because of the nuts.

Next, place cooked quinoa in a glass bowl and add in the pesto you just made. Mix them together until the pesto is evenly distributed throughout the quinoa. Add in the cooked butternut squash and toss everything together. You can serve this with a wedge of avocado and some basil. Enjoy.

Fried Rice

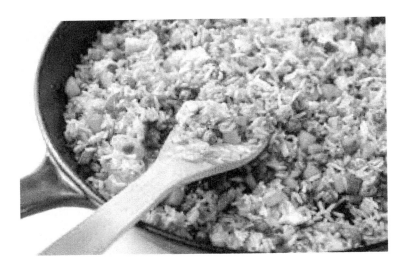

Preparation Time: 10 minutes

Cooking Time: 50 minutes

Serves: 3

Ingredients:

Cayenne pepper, to taste

Sea salt, to taste

Grapeseed oil, 1 tbsp

Diced onion, .25

Sliced zucchini, .5 c

Sliced mushrooms, .5 c

Sliced bell peppers, .5 c

Cooked quinoa or wild rice, 1 c

Instructions:

Place a skillet on top of stove and warm grapeseed oil. Add onion and cook until slightly browned and softened.

To the skillet, put all the other veggies and cook these for five more minutes. They should be soft but not mushy.

Add rice, stir to combine, and cook until slightly browned.

Green Vegetable Diet

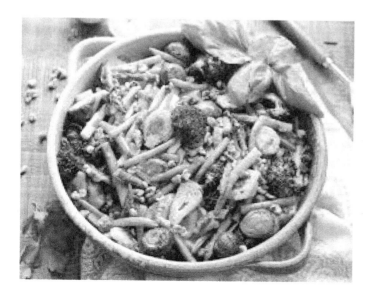

Preparation Time: 10 minutes

Cooking Time: 30 minutes

Serves: 3

Ingredients

Four cups of sliced Onions.

Six bunches of Mustard and T urnips greens.

Four tbsp of Sea salt.

Two tbsp of Olive oil.

Two tsp of Chili powder.

Instructions:

Place your fry pan on a source of heat.

Add Olive oil and allow heating.

Add onion and stir fry.

Add the green vegetables and simmer for 15 minutes or until done.

Add Chili powder and sea salt.

Taquitos Made with Mushroom

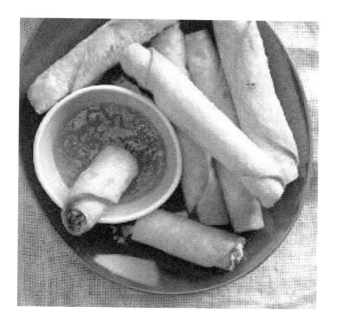

Preparation Time: 10 minutes

Cooking Time: 40 minutes

Serves: 3

Ingredients

Two tsp of ground Thyme.

Four tsp of chili powder.

Six tbsp of Sea salt.

Four tbsp of Oregano.

Four cups of sliced Onions.

Eight cups of sliced Mushrooms.

Four tbsp of Tomato sauce.

Four tsp of Onion powder.

Instructions:

Place a fry pan on a source of heat.

Add Olive oil and heat.

Add Onion stir fry until golden brown.

Add Mushroom and stir fry for 4 minutes.

Complement with seasonings.

Place in corn shells firmly.

Then fry until crunchy.

Veggie Pizza

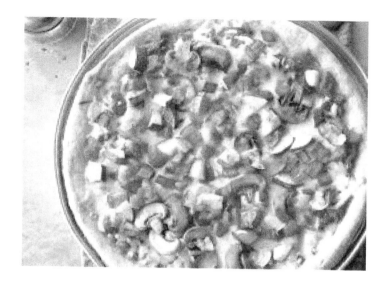

Preparation Time: 10 minutes

Cooking Time: 50 minutes

Serves: 3

Ingredients:

Alkaline Pizza Crust – recipe found in next section

Brazil nut cheese

Red bell peppers

Green bell peppers

Onion

Tomatoes

Avocado

Mushrooms

Oregano

Tomato Pizza Sauce:

Basil

Grapeseed oil, 2 tbsp

Oregano, 1 tsp.

Agave, 2 tbsp

Sea salt, 1 tsp.

Chopped onion, 2 tbsp

Roma tomatoes, 5

Onion powder, 1 tsp.

Avocado Pizza Sauce:

Basil

Onion powder, .5 tsp.

Chopped onion, 2 tbsp

Oregano, .5 tsp.

Avocado

Sea salt, .5 tsp.

Instructions:

First, let's make the two pizza sauces. For the tomato sauce, start by making small x-shaped cuts on both ends of the tomatoes and then place them into some boiling water. Only let them boil for a minute.

Immediately remove the tomato from the boiling water and put it into an ice bath for 30 seconds. The skin should easily peel off. Place your prepared tomatoes into a blender along with the other tomato sauce ingredients. Blend everything together until combined.

For the avocado sauce, slice the avocado in half and take out the pit. Scrape all of the insides into your food processor. Put the remaining sauce ingredients and blend about three minutes, or until it becomes smooth.

Now let's prepare the pizza. Take your flatbread pizza crust and spread one half with the tomato sauce and the other half with the avocado sauce. Sprinkle the Brazil nut cheese over the pizza and then add what approved toppings you would like.

Make sure that your oven is warmed to 400 and then bake your pizza for 15 to 20 minutes. Enjoy.

Rice and Spinach Balls

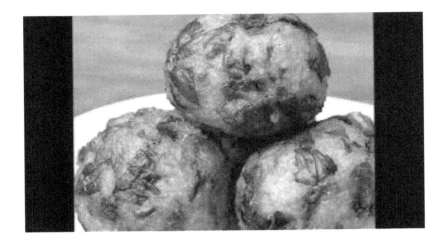

Preparation Time: 10 minutes

Cooking Time: 30 minutes

Serves: 3

Ingredients:

For Part One

Juice of one key lime

Pitted Greek olives, .33 c

Sea salt, .75 tsp.

Spinach leaves, 4.5 c

Onion powder, 1 tsp.

For Part Two

Chickpea flour, .5 c

Ground almonds, .5 c

Cooked wild rice, 1.25 c

Instructions:

Warm your oven to 360. Place all the ingredients for part one into either a food processor or a blender whichever one you have access to. Turn on the device until everything is well combined.

Add this mixture to a large bowl and add in all the ingredients for part two. Mix this together until it forms a dough. If it seems too wet, add some more flour. You can add in some cayenne pepper for taste if you would like. I don't recommend that you taste this as chickpea flour can be very bitter.

Take this mixture and scoop it out with a spoon. Roll it in between your palms until it turns into a ball. Place these onto a cookie sheet that has parchment paper on it. This should make one dozen balls. Place into the oven for 20 minutes. If you want to check for doneness, you will have to taste one of them. Be careful not to burn your mouth. If you don't taste any bitterness, they are done.

Roasted Vegetables

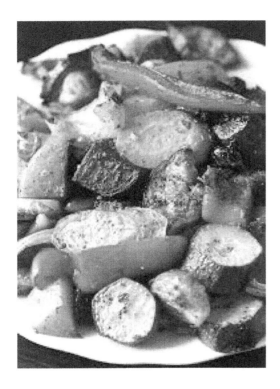

Preparation Time: 10 minutes

Cooking Time: 15 minutes

Serves: 2

Ingredients:

1-pint cherry tomatoes

2 cups chopped asparagus

1/2 cup halved mushrooms

1 tsp. sea salt

1 tbsp. onion powder

1 tbsp. coconut oil

1 seeded and chopped red bell pepper

1 peeled zucchini, cut into small bite-size pieces

Instructions:

Adjust the temperature of your oven to 425° F.

In a bowl, mix all of the ingredients as you evenly coat the vegetables.

Transfer the vegetables into a baking pan.

Roast the vegetables for about 15 minutes until the vegetables are tender.

Serve.

Curried Zucchini

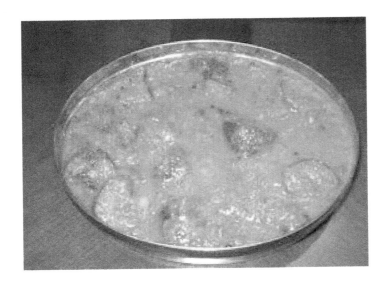

Preparation Time: 5 minutes

Cooking Time: 5 minutes

Serves: 2

Ingredients:

Cooked quinoa

Flesh roasted zucchini

Water

1 tsp. curry powder

1 tsp. sea salt

1 tsp. sesame oil

1 seville orange juice

Instructions:

In the food processor, mix the salt, zucchini, sesame oil, seville orange juice, and curry powder.

Blend the mixture until it becomes smooth.

In a saucepan over moderate heat, transfer zucchini mixture then warm it for 5 minutes.

Add a little water to thin it.

Serve over the cooked quinoa.

Serve.

Mushrooms and Rice

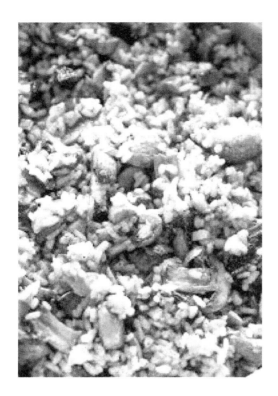

Preparation Time: 10 minutes

Cooking Time: 30 minutes

Serves: 3

Ingredients:

1 cup of mushrooms, chopped

1 cup of wild rice, cooked

½ cup kale

1 teaspoon olive oil

1 teaspoon of sea salt

Instructions:

Cook kale and rice independently. Leave them to cool.

Prepare mushrooms (they can be cooked, baked or barbecued).

Top mushrooms with oil and salt. Serve with kale and rice.

Sautéed Radish

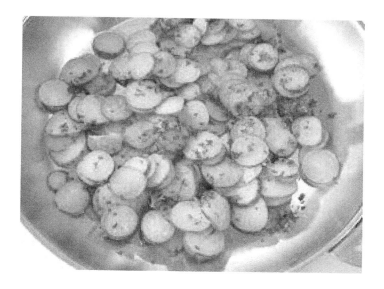

Preparation Time: 5 minutes

Cooking Time: 10 minutes

Serves: 2

Ingredients:

1/2 cup light sweetened coconut milk

1-1/2 tsps. ground ginger

1 tsp. freshly squeezed lime juice

1/2 tsp. chili-chive sauce

1 tbsp. coconut oil

1/2 tsp. sea salt

3/4 lb. trimmed and halved Radish with ends removed

1 packet Stevia

Instructions:

In a saucepan over moderate heat, mix the ground ginger, coconut milk, lime juice, chili-chive sauce, and Stevia.

Allow it to simmer.

Cook for 5 minutes then remove the pan from the heat.

Set it aside.

In a separate bowl, add the Radish, sea salt, and the coconut oil then toss them to mix.

Transfer the Radish mixture into ovenproof skillet or an iron pan.

Sauté the Brussels over moderate heat for 5 minutes.

Preheat the broiler.

Place the Raddish in the boiler then boil it for 3 minutes until the leaves become slightly brown.

Transfer the Radish to the serving bowls.

You can add the sauce then toss to coat it.

Serve.

Chapter 13: Sauces Recipes

Tomato Pizza Sauce

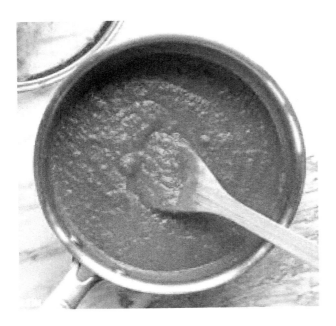

Preparation Time: 10 minutes

Cooking Time: 0 minutes

Serves: 3

Ingredients

1 tsp. Onion Powder

2 tbsp. Agave

5 Roma Tomatoes

2 tbsp of chopped Onion

pinch of Basil

1 tsp. Sea Salt

1 tsp. Oregano

2 tbsp. Grape Seed Oil

Instructions

Make small x-looking cuts on the edges of five plum tomatoes to remove the skin, and place in boiling water for a minute.

Place the tomatoes in cold water for 40 seconds so you can easily peel the skin.

Blend the tomatoes and the other ingredients until smooth.

Spaghetti Squash with Tomato Sauce

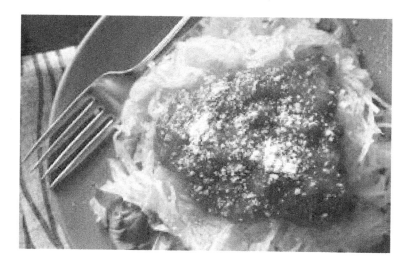

Preparation Time: 15 minutes

Cooking Time: 0 minutes

Serves: 2

Ingredients:

1 tsp. minced chive

1 tsp. sea salt

1 tsp. coconut oil

1/4 chopped onion

1/2 tsp. red pepper flakes

2 cups shredded cooked spaghetti squash

1/2 cup water

16 oz. can tomato paste

Instructions:

In a pot over moderate heat, sauté the onions in the coconut oil for 5 minutes until it becomes tender.

Add the tomato paste, salt, red pepper flakes, and chive the stir properly to mix.

Add the spaghetti sauce and water.

Simmer the meal for 10 minutes.

Add in the spaghetti squash then stir properly to mix them.

Serve.

Zoodles in Avocado Sauce

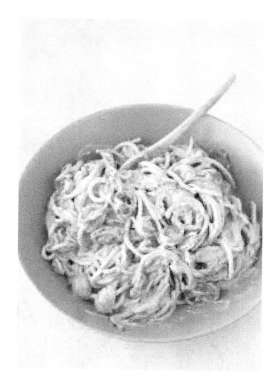

Preparation Time: 10 minutes

Cooking Time: 0 minutes

Serves: 3

Ingredients:

Sea salt, to taste

Cherry tomatoes, 24 sliced

Avocados, 2

Key lime juice, 4 tbsp

Walnuts, .5 c

Water, .5 c

Basil, 2 c

Zucchinis, 2 large

Instructions:

You will need to make the zoodles by either using a spiralizer or a peeler.

Place salt, avocados, lime juice, walnuts, and basil into a blender and process until creamy.

Place the zoodles into a bowl. Add tomatoes, avocado sauce, and zoodles. Toss until well coated. Enjoy.

Chapter 14: Special Ingredients Recipes

Stomach Soother

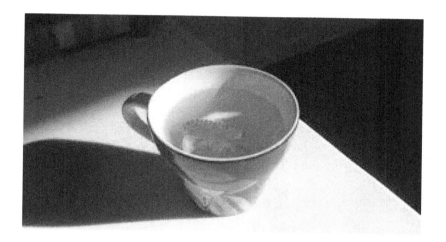

Preparation Time: 10 minutes

Cooking Time: 0 minutes

Serves: 3

Ingredients:

Agave syrup, 1 tbsp

Ginger tea, .5 c

Dr. Sebi's Stomach Relief Herbal Tea

Burro banana, 1

Instructions:

Fix the herbal tea according to the directions on the package. Set it aside to cool.

Once the tea is cool, place it along with all the other ingredients into a blender. Turn the blender on and let it run until it is creamy.

Sarsaparilla Syrup

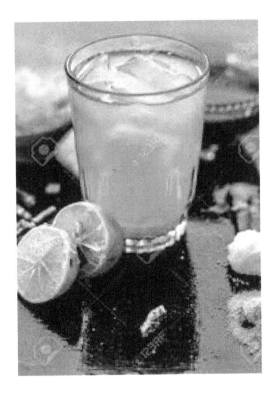

Preparation Time: 10 minutes

Cooking Time: 0 minutes

Serves: 3

Ingredients:

Date sugar, 1 c

Sassafras root, 1 tbsp

Sarsaparilla root, 1 c

Water, 2 c

Instructions:

Start by adding all of the ingredients to a mason jar. Screw on the lid, tightly, and shake everything together. Heat a water bath up to 160. Sit the mason jar into the water bath and allow it to infuse for about two to four hours.

When the infusion time is almost up, set up an ice bath. Add half and half water and ice to a bowl. Carefully take the mason jar out of the water bath and place it into the ice bath. Allow it to sit in the ice bath for 15 to 20 minutes.

Strain the infusion out and into another clean jar. This will last for at least a week when kept in the refrigerator.

Dandelion "Coffee"

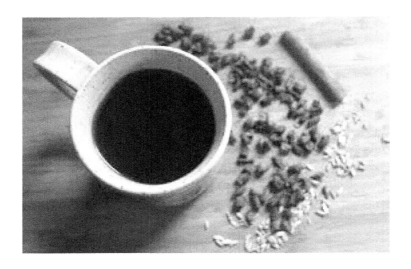

Preparation Time: 10 minutes

Cooking Time: 30 minutes

Serves: 3

Ingredients:

Nettle leaf, a pinch

Roasted dandelion root, 1 t bsp

Water, 24 oz

Instructions:

To start, we will roast the dandelion root to help bring out its flavors. Feel free to use raw dandelion root if you want to, but roasted root brings out an earthy and complex flavor, which is perfect for cool mornings.

Simply add the dandelion root to a pre-warmed cast iron skillet. Allow the pieces to roast on medium heat until they start to darken in color, and you

140

start to smell their rich aroma. Make sure that you don't let them burn because this will ruin your teas taste.

As the root is roasting, have the water in a pot and allow it to come up to a full, rapid boil. Once your dandelion is roasted, add it to the boiling water with the nettle leaf. Steep this for ten minutes.

Strain. You can flavor your tea with some agave if you want to. Enjoy.

Chamomile Delight

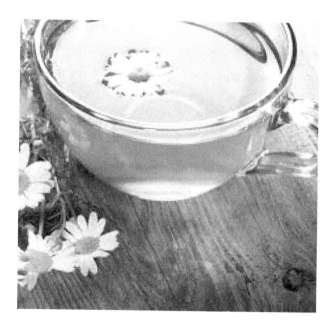

Preparation Time: 10 minutes

Cooking Time: 30 minutes

Serves: 3

Ingredients:

Date sugar, 1 tbsp

Walnut milk, .5 c

Dr. Sebi's Nerve/Stress Relief Herbal Tea, .25 c

Burro banana, 1

Instructions:

Prepare the tea according to the package directions. Set to the side and allow to cool.

Once the tea is cooled, add it along with the above ingredients to a blender and process until creamy and smooth.

Mucus Cleanse Tea

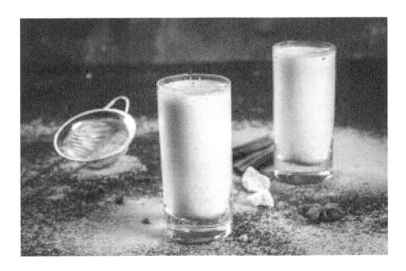

Preparation Time: 10 minutes
Cooking Time: 30 minutes

Serves: 3

Ingredients:

Blue Vervain

Bladderwrack

Irish Sea Moss

Instructions:

Add the sea moss to your blender. This would be best as a gel. Just make sure that it is totally dry.

Place equal parts of the bladder-wrack to the blender. Again, this would be best as a gel. Just make sure that it is totally dry. To get the best results you need to chop these by hand.

Add equal parts of the blue vervain to the blender. You can use the roots to increase your iron intake and nutritional healing values.

Process the herbs until they form a powder. This can take up to three minutes.

Place the powder into a non-metal pot and put it on the stove. Fill the pot half full of water. Make sure the herbs are totally immersed in water. Turn on the heat and let the liquid boil. Don't let it boil more than five minutes.

Carefully strain out the herbs. You can save these for later use in other recipes.

Let the liquid cool to your liking and enjoy.

You can add in some agave nectar, date sugar, or key lime juice for added flavor.

Immune Tea

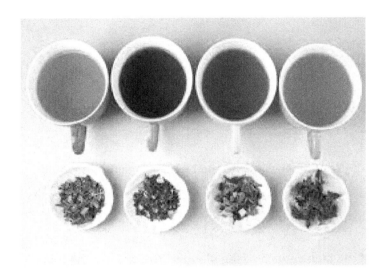

Preparation Time: 10 minutes

Cooking Time: 30 minutes

Serves: 3

Ingredients:

Echinacea, 1 part

Astragalus, 1 part

Rosehip, 1 part

Chamomile, 1 part

Elderflowers, 1 part

Elderberries, 1 part

Instructions:

Mix the herbs together and place them inside an airtight container.

When you are ready to make a cup of tea, place one teaspoon into a tea ball or bag, and put it in eight ounces of boiling water. Let this sit for 20 minutes.

Ginger Turmeric Tea

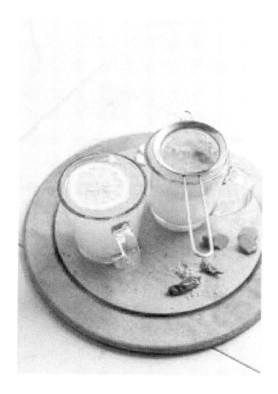

Preparation Time: 10 minutes

Cooking Time: 20 minutes

Serves: 3

Ingredients:

Juice of one key lime

Turmeric finger, couple of slices

Ginger root, couple of slices

Water, 3 c

Instructions:

Pour the water into a pot and let it boil. Remove from heat and put the turmeric and ginger in. Stir well. Place lid on pot and let it sit 15 minutes.

While you are waiting on your tea to finish steeping, juice one key lime, and divide between two mugs.

Once the tea is ready, remove the turmeric and ginger and pour the tea into mugs and enjoy. If you want your tea a bit sweet, add some agave syrup or date sugar.

Date Syrup

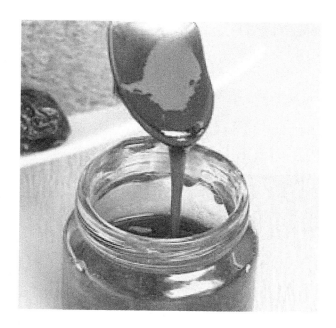

Preparation Time: 10 minutes

Cooking Time: 0 minutes

Serves: 3

Ingredients

1 cup dates, hollowed

1 cup spring water

Instructions:

1. Heat up spring water on burner, then remove from heat.

2. Sit dates in the water for 15 minutes.

3. Empty water and dates into blender and mix for 1 moment or until smooth.

4. If consistency is excessively thick, add around 1/4 cup of water and mix again.

5. Store in the fridge and make the most of your Alkaline Date Syrup!

Tranquil Tea

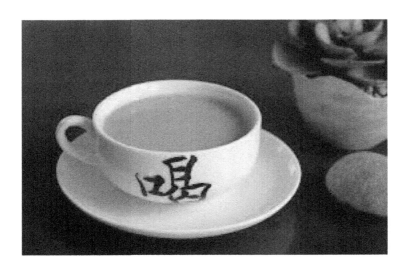

Preparation Time: 10 minutes

Cooking Time: 30 minutes

Serves: 3

Ingredients:

Rose petals, 2 parts

Lemongrass, 2 parts

Chamomile, 4 parts

Instructions:

Put all the herbs into a glass jar and shake well to mix.

When you are ready to make a cup of tea, add one teaspoon of the mixture for every serving to a tea strainer, ball, or bag. Cover with water that has boiled and let it sit for ten minutes.

If you like a little sweetness in your tea, you can add some agave syrup or date sugar.

Energizing Lemon Tea

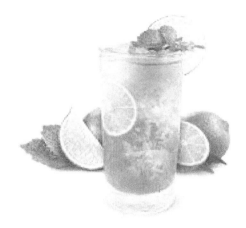

Preparation Time: 10 minutes

Cooking Time: 10 minutes

Serves: 3

Ingredients:

Lemongrass, .5 tsp. dried herb

Lemon thyme, .5 tsp. dried herb

Lemon verbena, 1 tsp. dried herb

Instructions:

Place the dried herbs into a tea strainer, bag, or ball and place it in one cup of water that has boiled. Let this sit 15 minutes. Carefully strain out the tea. You can add agave syrup or date sugar if needed.

Quick note: If your herbs are fresh, you just need to triple the amounts above.

Respiratory Support Tea

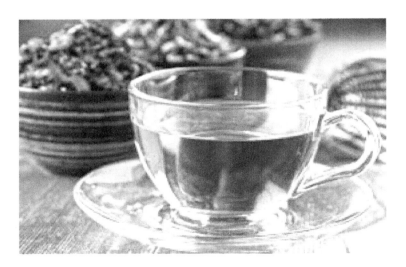

Preparation Time: 10 minutes

Cooking Time: 20 minutes

Serves: 3

Ingredients:

Rosehip, 2 parts

Lemon balm, 1 part

Coltsfoot leaves, 1 part

Mullein, 1 part

Osha root, 1 part

Marshmallow root, 1 part

Instructions:

Place three cups of water into a pot. Place the Osha root and marshmallow root into the pot. Allow to boil. Let this simmer for ten minutes Now put the remaining ingredients into the pot and let this steep another eight minutes. Strain. Drink three to four cups of this tea each day.

It's almost that time of year again when everyone is suffering from the dreaded cold. Then that cold turns into a nasty lingering cough. Having these ingredients on hand will help you be able to get ahead of this year's cold season. When you buy your ingredient, they need to be stored in glass jars. The roots and leaves need to be put into separate jars. You can drink this tea at any time, but it is great for when you need some extra respiratory support.

Chapter 15: Snacks & Bread Recipes

Pumpkin Spice Crackers

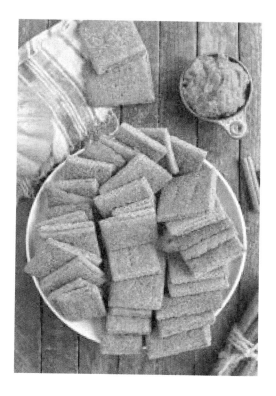

Preparation Time: 10 minutes

Cooking Time: 1 hr.

Serves: 6

Ingredients:

1/3 cup coconut flour

2 tbsps. pumpkin pie spice

3/4 cup sunflower seeds

3/4 cup flaxseed

1/3 cup sesame seeds

1 tbsp. ground psyllium husk powder

1 tsp. sea salt

3 tbsps. melted coconut oil

1-1/3 cups alkaline water

Instructions:

Adjust the temperature of your oven to 300ºF.

In a bowl, mix all the dry ingredients.

Add the water and oil to the mixture then properly mix it.

Let the dough settle for about 3 mins.

You then spread the dough on a cookie sheet lined with parchment paper.

Bake for about 30 minutes.

Reduce the temperature of the oven then bake for an extra 30 minutes.

Crack the bread into bite-size pieces.

Serve.

Spicy Roasted Nuts

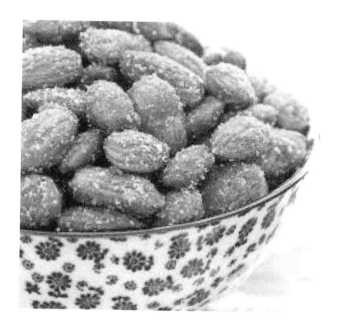

Preparation Time: 10 minutes

Cooking Time: 15 minutes

Serves: 4

Ingredients:

8 oz. walnuts

1 tsp. sea salt

1 tsp. coconut oil

1 tsp. cumin, ground

1 tsp. powdered paprika

Instructions:

Place all the ingredients in a skillet.

Roast the nuts until they turn golden brown.

Serve and enjoy.

Potato Chips

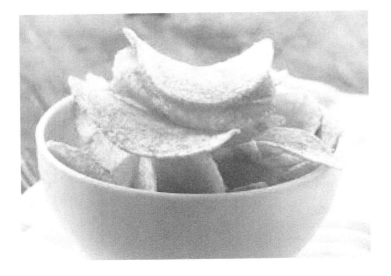

Preparation Time: 10 minutes

Cooking Time: 5 minutes

Serves: 4

Ingredients:

1 tbsp. vegetable oil

1 sliced paper-thin potato

Sea salt

Instructions:

Place the potato with the oil and sea salt.

Spread the slices in a baking dish in a single layer.

Cook the meal in a microwave for about 5 minutes until golden brown.

Serve.

Zucchini Pepper Chips

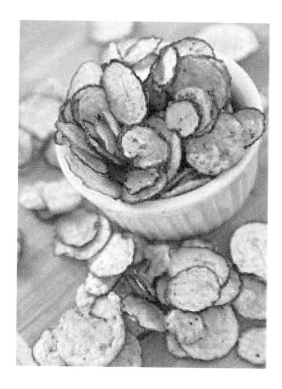

Preparation Time: 10 minutes

Cooking Time: 15 minutes

Serves: 4

Ingredients:

1-2/3 cups vegetable oil

2 zucchinis, thinly sliced

1 tsp. onion powder

1/2 tsp. ground black pepper

3 tbsps. red pepper flakes, crushed

Instructions:

Mix the oil with all the spices in a bowl.

Then add the zucchini slices and mix well.

Transfer the mixture to a Ziplock bag then seal it.

Refrigerate the mixture for about 10 minutes.

Spread the zucchini slices on a greased baking sheet.

Bake for about 15 minutes.

Serve.

Onion Rings

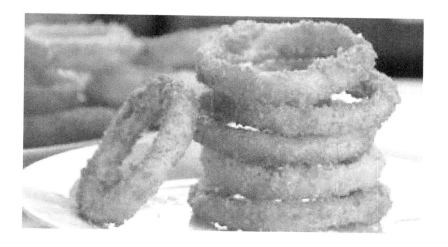

Preparation Time: 6 minutes

Cooking Time: 30 minutes

Serving: 8

Ingredients:

Peeled and sliced White Onions

1 cup Spelt Flour

1/2 cup Homemade Hempseed Milk

1/2 cup Aquafaba

2 tsps. Onion Powder

2 tsps. Oregano

1 tsp. Cayenne Powder

2 tsps. Pure Sea Salt

3 tbsps. Grape Seed Oil

Instructions:

Adjust the temperature of your oven to 450ºF.

Pour Homemade Hempseed Milk and the Aquafaba into a bowl then whisk them properly.

Add 1 tsp. of Oregano, 1 tsp. of Onion Powder, 1/2 tsp. of Cayenne, and 1 tsp. of Pure Sea Salt to the wet ingredients then mix.

Separate the onion slices into rings.

Add the Spelt Flour, 1 tsp. of Oregano, 1 tsp. of Onion Powder, 1/2 tsp. of Cayenne, and 1 tsp. of Pure Sea Salt to a container with a lid.

Shake all the dry ingredients properly.

Brush a baking sheet with the Grape Seed Oil

Place a few of the onion rings in the wet mixture.

Put wet onion rings in the dry mixture then flip until they get coated on both sides

Put the covered onion rings on the baking sheet.

Repeat the procedure 8 through 10 until all onion rings are covered.

Lightly drizzle the rings with Grape Seed Oil.

Bake for about 15 minutes until golden brown.

Allow the meal to cool.

Serve and enjoy.

Flatbread

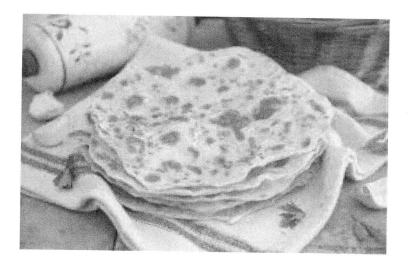

Preparation Time: 5 minutes

Cooking Time: 20 minutes

Serving: 3

Ingredients:

Sea salt, 1 tbsp

Cayenne, .25 tsp.

Oregano, 2 tsp.

Springwater, .75 c

Onion powder, 2 tsp.

Grapeseed oil, 2 tbsp

Basil, 2 tsp.

Instructions:

Combine the seasonings together into the flour. Stir in the oil and mix in a half cup of the water.

Slowly add in the rest of the water until the dough forms a ball.

Sprinkle some flour over your workspace and then knead your dough for five minutes. Divide it into six parts.

Roll the balls into four-inch circles.

Lay them out on an ungreased skillet that has been heated to medium-high. Flip it every two to three minutes, or until it is cooked through. Enjoy.

Sloppy Joe

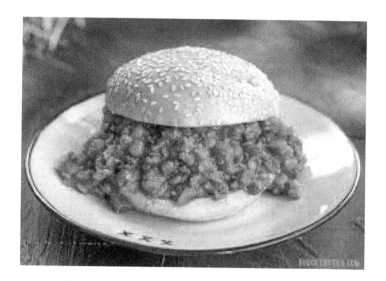

Preparation Time: 5 minutes

Cooking Time: 30 minutes

Serving: 3

Ingredients:

Grapeseed oil

Cayenne pepper, pinch

Sea salt, 1 tsp.

Diced plum tomato

Onion powder, 1 tsp.

Diced green bell peppers, .5 c

Diced onion, .5 c

Cooked garbanzo beans, 1 c

Barbecue sauce, 1.5 c

Cooked Kamut or spelt, 2 c

Barbecue Sauce:

Cloves, pinch

Onion powder, 2 tsp.

Cayenne, .25 tsp.

Ground ginger, .5 tsp.

Sea salt, 2 tsp.

Chopped white onions, .25 c

Date sugar, .25 c

Agave nectar, 2 tbsp

Plum tomatoes, 6

Instructions:

Let's begin by making the barbecue sauce. Add all of the barbecue sauce ingredients, minus the date sugar, to your blender and mix together until smooth and combined.

Pour all of the blended ingredients into a pot along with the date sugar. Allow the mixture to heat up until it comes to a boil. Make sure you occasionally stir it. Turn the heat down and allow it to simmer, covered, for about 15 minutes. Stir it occasionally as it cooks.

To make the sauce smoother, you can use an immersion blender at this point. With the lid off, and simmering, allow it to cook for about ten minutes more or until the water has cooked off. Let the sauce cool completely. It will thicken as it cools.

Next, add the garbanzo beans and spelt to a food processor and pulse it together for about ten to 15 seconds. Place some oil into a large skillet and add in the peppers, onions, and seasonings and sauté everything for about three to five minutes.

Stir in the pulsed ingredients, barbecue sauce, and tomato. Allow this all to simmer together for another five minutes. This is great served with some alkaline flatbread.

Apple Chips

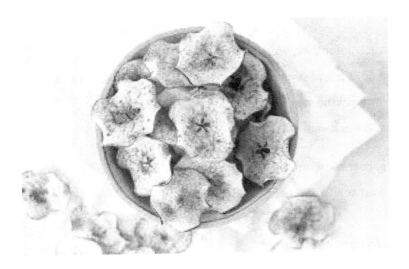

Preparation Time: 5 minutes

Cooking Time: 45 minutes

Serves: 4

Ingredients:

2 cored and thinly sliced Golden Delicious apples

1-1/2 tsps. date sugar

1/2 tsp. ground cinnamon

Instructions:

Adjust the temperature of oven to 225ºF.

Put the apple slices on a baking sheet.

Sprinkle the sugar on the apples.

Add cinnamon over apple slices.

Bake for about 45 minutes.

Serve.

Kale Crisps

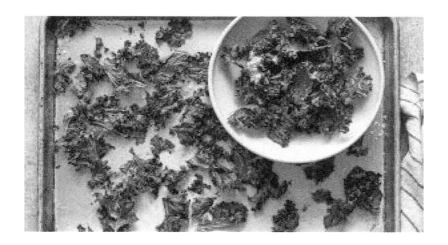

Preparation Time: 10 minutes

Cooking Time: 10 minutes

Serves: 4

Ingredients:

1 bunch kale with stems removed, leaves torn into even pieces

1 tbsp. olive oil

1 tsp. sea salt

Instructions:

Adjust the temperature of your oven to 350ºF.

Layer a baking sheet with parchment paper.

Spread the kale leaves on a paper towel to absorb the moisture.

Add salt and olive oil to the leaves.

Spread them on the baking sheet then bake for about 10 minutes.

Serve.

Zucchini Chips

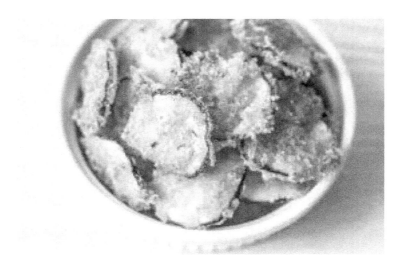

Preparation Time: 5 minutes

Cooking Time: 12 minutes

Serves: 4

Ingredients:

4 washed, peeled and sliced zucchinis

2 tsps. extra-virgin olive oil

1/4 tsp. sea salt

Instructions:

Adjust the temperature of your oven to 350ºF.

Add salt and the olive oil to the zucchinis.

Spread the slices on two baking sheets in a single layer.

Bake for about 6 minutes on both the upper and lower rack of the oven.

Switch the baking racks and bake for an extra 6 minutes.

Serve.

Turnip Chips

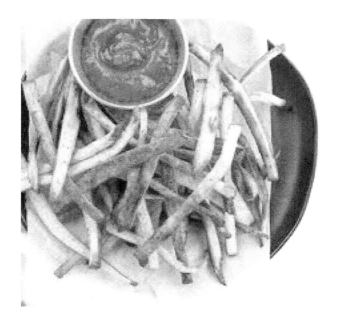

Preparation Time: 5 minutes

Cooking Time: 5 minutes

Serves: 4

Ingredients:

1 thinly sliced turnip

2 tsps. olive oil

Coarse sea salt

Instructions:

Toss the turnip with oil and salt.

Spread the slices in a baking dish in a single layer.

Cook in a microwave for about 5 minutes until golden brown.

Serve.

Chapter 16: Desserts Recipes

Blueberry Muffins

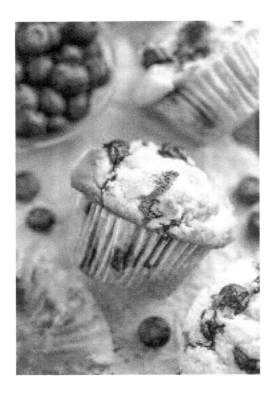

Preparation Time: 5 minutes

Cooking Time: 20 minutes

Serving: 3

Ingredients:

Grapeseed oil

Sea salt, .5 tsp.

Sea moss gel, .25 c

Agave, .3 c

Blueberries, .5 c

Teff flour, .75 c

Spelt flour, .75 c

Coconut milk, 1 c

Instructions:

Warm your oven to 365. Place paper liners into a muffin tin.

Place sea moss gel, sea salt, agave, flour, and milk in large bowl. Mix well to combine. Gently fold in blueberries.

Gently pour batter into paper liners. Place in oven and bake 30 minutes.

They are done when they have turned a nice golden color, and they spring back when you touch them.

Brazil Nut Cheese

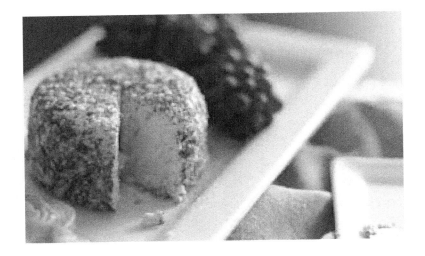

Preparation Time: 5 minutes

Cooking Time: 20 minutes

Serving: 3

Ingredients:

Grapeseed oil, 2 tsp.

Water, 1.5 c

Hemp milk, 1.5 c

Cayenne, .5 tsp.

Onion powder, 1 tsp.

Juice of .5 lime

Sea salt, 2 tsp.

Brazil nuts, 1 lb.

Onion powder, 1 tsp.

Instructions:

You will need to start by soaking the Brazil nuts in some water. You just put the nuts into a bowl and make sure the water covers them. Soak no less than two hours or overnight. Overnight would be best.

Now you need to put everything except water into a food processor or blender.

Add just .5 cups water and blend for two minutes

Continue adding .5 cup water and blending until you have the consistency you want.

Scrape into an airtight container and enjoy.

Baked Stuffed Pears

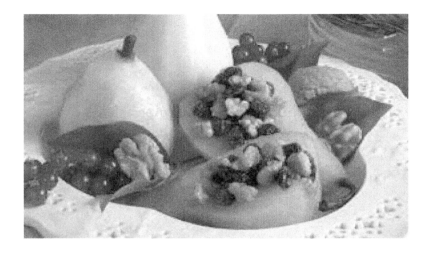

Preparation Time: 5 minutes

Cooking Time: 20 minutes

Serving: 3

Ingredients:

Agave syrup, 4 tbsp

Cloves, .25 tsp.

Chopped walnuts, 4 tbsp

Currants, 1 c

Pears, 4

Instructions:

Make sure your oven has been warmed to 375.

Slice the pears in two lengthwise and remove the core. To get the pear to lay flat, you can slice a small piece off the back side.

Place the agave syrup, currants, walnuts, and cloves in a small bowl and mix well. Set this to the side to be used later.

Put the pears on a cookie sheet that has parchment paper on it. Make sure the cored sides are facing up. Sprinkle each pear half with about .5 tablespoon of the chopped walnut mixture.

Place into the oven and cook for 25 to 30 minutes. Pears should be tender.

Dr. Sebi strawberry banana ice cream recipe

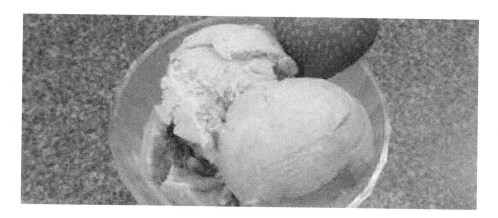

Preparation Time: 5 minutes

Cooking Time: 0 minutes

Serving: 3

Ingredients

1 cup frozen strawberries

1 tbsp. Agave

1/4 cup Nut/Hemp Milk Blender

5 Frozen Baby Bananas

1/2 of Avocado Frozen fruits is optional but it will allow the ice cream set faster if you use it.

Direction

1. Grab your blender, toss in all the ingredients then blend until well mixed.

2. Take a pinch out of the ingredients then taste for sweetness and texture. Add more agave if it needs more sweetness or more milk if it is too thick.

3. Scoop into an air-tight container and freeze for 6 hours until its firm.

4. Your ice cream is ready to be scooped and served.

Alkaline-Electric Ice Cream

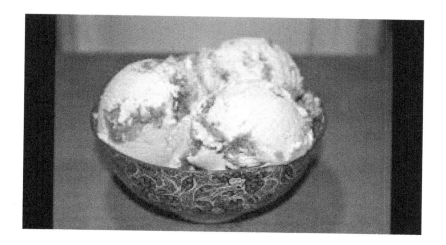

Preparation Time: 5 minutes

Cooking Time: 20 minutes

Serving: 3

Ingredients

Agave syrup

3 tablespoons of homemade walnut milk

2 ripe mangoes

2 burro bananas

Instructions

Peel and then cut all your mangoes into small cubes.

Peel and slice the burro bananas.

Put both the banana mango and pieces in a baking sheet lined with parchment paper and freeze.

Place your frozen fruit in a food processor and add the sweetener and the homemade walnut milk.

Blend for 4 minutes.

You need to stop it throughout to push it down and stir it around.

Serve and enjoy.

Strawberry Sorbet

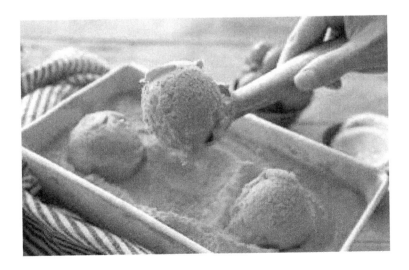

Preparation Time: 5 minutes

Cooking Time: 4 hours

Serves: 4

Ingredients

2 cups Strawberries

1 1/2 tsps. Spelt Flour

1/2 cup Date Sugar

2 cups Spring Water

Instructions:

Add the Date Sugar, Spelt Flour, and Spring Water to a pot then boil on low heat for about 10 minutes until the mixture gets thick.

Remove the pot from the heat then allow it to cool.

After it has cooled, add the Strawberry then mix gently.

Place the mixture in a container then freeze.

Cut it into pieces, put the sorbet into a processor and blend until smooth.

Put everything back in the container and leave in the refrigerator for at least 4 hours.

Serve and enjoy.

Banana Strawberry Ice Cream

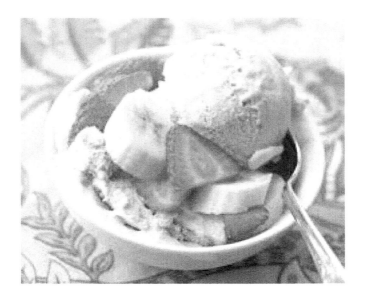

Preparation Time: 10 minutes

Cooking Time: 0 minutes

Serves: 5

Ingredients:

1 cup Strawberry

5 quartered Baby Bananas

1/2 chopped Avocado

1 tbsp. Agave Syrup

1/4 cup Homemade Walnut Milk

Instructions:

Place all the ingredients into the blender then blend them properly.

Taste it. If it is too thick, add extra Milk or the Agave Syrup if you want it sweeter.

Then place it in a container with a lid and allow it to freeze for at least 6 hours.

Serve and enjoy.

Homemade Whipped Cream

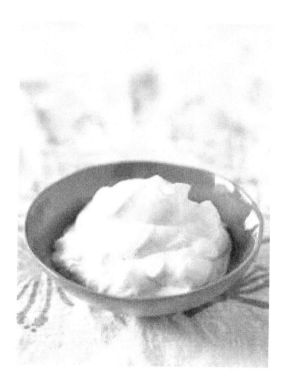

Preparation Time: 5 minutes

Cooking Time: 0 minutes

Serves: 1

Ingredients:

1 cup Aquafaba

1/4 cup Agave Syrup

Instructions:

Add the Agave Syrup and the Aquafaba to a bowl.

Mix using a stand mixer at high speed for about 5 minutes then using a hand mixer for about 15 minutes.

Serve and enjoy.

Chocolate Pudding

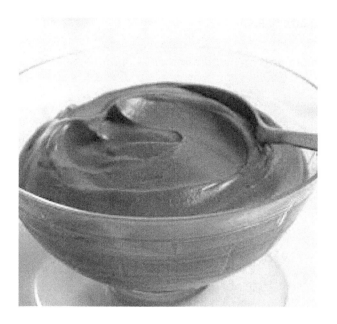

Preparation Time: 5 minutes

Cooking Time: 0 minutes

Serves: 4

Ingredients:

2 cups seedless Black Sapote

1/4 cup Agave Syrup

1/2 cup-soaked Brazil Nuts

1 tbsp. Hemp Seeds

1/2 cup Spring Water

Instructions:

Cut 2 cups of Black Sapote into half.

Put all ingredients into a blender then blend them until smooth.

Serve and enjoy.

Butternut Squash Pie

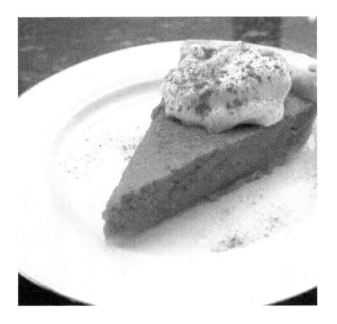

Preparation Time: 5 minutes

Cooking Time: 20 minutes

Serves: 4

Ingredients:

For the Crust

Cold water

Agave, splash

Sea salt, pinch

Grapeseed oil, .5 c

Coconut flour, .5 c

Spelt Flour, 1 c

For the Filling

Butternut squash, peeled, chopped

Water

Allspice, to taste

Agave syrup, to taste

Hemp milk, 1 c

Sea moss, 4 tbsp

Instructions:

You will need to warm your oven to 350.

For the Crust

Place the grapeseed oil and water into the refrigerator to get it cold. This will take about one hour.

Place all ingredients into a large bowl. Now you need to add in the cold water a little bit in small amounts until a dough form. Place this onto a surface that has been sprinkled with some coconut flour. Knead for a few minutes and roll the dough as thin as you can get it. Carefully pick it up and place it inside a pie plate.

Place the butternut squash into a Dutch oven and pour in enough water to cover. Bring this to a full rolling boil. Let this cook until the squash has become soft.

Completely drain and place into bowl. Using a potato masher, mash the squash. Add in some allspice and agave to taste. Add in the sea moss and hemp milk. Using a hand mixer, blend well. Pour into the pie crust.

Place into the oven and bake for about one hour.

Cheesecake

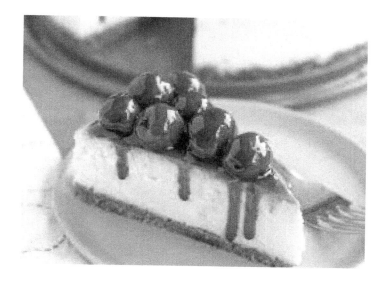

Preparation Time: 5 minutes

Cooking Time: 30 minutes

Serves: 4

Ingredients

Cheesecake:

Sea salt, .25 tsp.

Sea moss gel, 1 tbsp

Lime juice, 2 tbsp

Dates, 5 to 6

Agave, .25 c

Hemp or walnut milk, 1.5 c

Brazil nuts, 2 c

Crust:

Sea salt, .25 tsp.

Agave, .25 c

Coconut flakes, 1.5 c

Dates, 1.5 c

Topping:

Blackberries

Blueberries

Sliced raspberries

Sliced strawberry

Sliced mango

Instructions:

Add all of the crust ingredients into your food processor and blend it for about 20 seconds.

Spread your crust out into a springform pan that has been covered with parchment.

Place the mango slices along the side of the pan and then place it in the freezer as you prepare everything else.

Add everything for the cheesecake to your blender and mix it together until it creates a smooth mixture.

Remove the springform pan from the freezer and pour the filling in. Wrap in foil and let it sit for three to four hours.

Carefully remove from the pan, and then place the rest of the toppings over the top. All of the leftovers should be kept in the freezer.

Banana Cream Pie

Preparation Time: 5 minutes

Cooking Time: 20 minutes

Serves: 4

Ingredients:

Filling:

Sea salt, pinch

Agave, 3 to 4 tbsp

Hemp milk, 1 c

Creamed coconut, 7 oz

Baby bananas, 6 to 8

Crust:

Sea salt, .25 tsp.

Agave, .25 c

Unsweetened coconut flakes, 1.5 c

Pitted dates, 1.5 c

Instructions:

Add the crust ingredients to your food processor and mix it until it creates a ball.

Add some parchment paper to your springform pan. Spread your crust evenly across the pan.

Thinly slice the bananas and lay them along the inside of the pan. Place it in the freezer.

Place the filling mixture into a bowl and use an electric mixer to mix it all together.

Pour the filling into the pan. Shake the pan to even out the filling. Cover the pan with the foil and place it back in the freezer for three to four hours.

Top the cake with coconut and enjoy.

Chapter 17: Smoothies Recipes

Detox berry smoothie

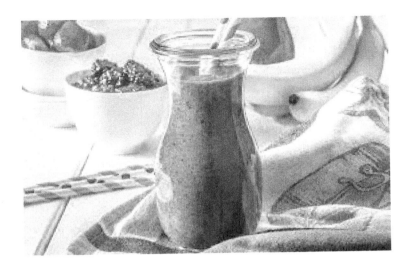

Preparation Time: 15 minutes

Cooking Time: 0 minutes

Serves: 1

Ingredients

Spring water

1/4 avocado, pitted

One medium burro banana

One seville orange

Two cups of fresh lettuce

One tablespoon of hemp seeds

One cup of berries (blueberries or an aggregate of blueberries, strawberries, and raspberries)

Instructions:

Add the spring water to your blender.

Put the fruits and vegies right inside the blender.

Blend all ingredients till smooth.

Apple and amaranth detoxifying smoothie

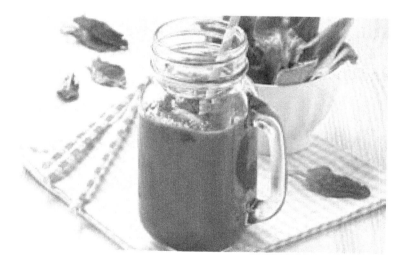

Preparation Time: 15 minutes

Cooking Time: 0 minutes

Serves: 1

Ingredients

1/4 avocado

1 key lime

Two apples, chopped

Two cups of water

Two cups of amaranth vegie

Instructions:

Put all the ingredients collectively in a blender

Blend all the ingredients evenly

Enjoy this delicious smoothie

Arugula and Cucumber Smoothie

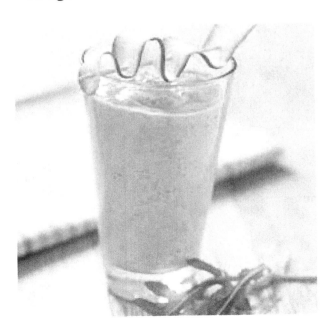

Preparation Time: 15 minutes

Cooking Time: 0 minutes

Serves: 1

Ingredients

2 cups of spring water

1 large bunch of callaloo, fresh

¼ cup of lime juice

1 cup diced cucumber, fresh

1 large bunch of arugula, fresh

¼ of a honeydew, fresh

1-inch piece of ginger, fresh

1 pear, destemmed, diced

6 Medjool dates, pitted

1 tablespoon of sea moss gel

Instructions:

Take a high-powered blender, switch it on, and then place all the ingredients inside, in order.

Cover the blender with its lid and then pulse at high speed for 1 minute or more until

Dandelion and Watercress Smoothie

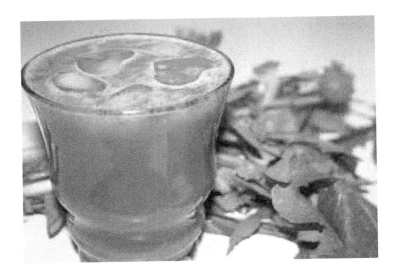

Preparation Time: 5 minutes

Cooking Time: 0 minutes

Serves: 1

Serves: 2

Ingredients

2 cups spring water

1 large bunch of dandelion greens, fresh

¼ cup key lime juice

1 cup of watercress, fresh

3 baby bananas, peeled

½ cup fresh blueberries

1-inch piece of ginger, fresh

6 Medjool dates, pitted

1 tablespoon burdock root powder

Instructions:

Take a high-powered blender, switch it on, and then place all the ingredients inside, in order.

Cover the blender with its lid and then pulse at high speed for 1 minute or more until.

Triple Berry Smoothie

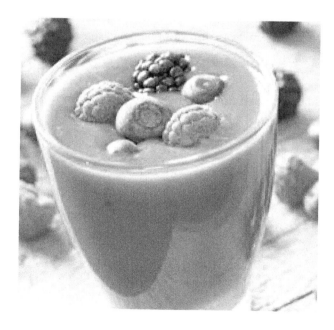

Preparation Time: 15 minutes

Cooking Time: 0 minutes

Serves: 1

Ingredients

1 cup spring water

1 cup fresh whole strawberries

2 small bananas

1 cup fresh whole raspberries

2 tablespoons agave syrup

1 cup fresh whole blueberries

Instructions:

Take a high-powered blender, switch it on, and then place all the ingredients inside, in order.

Cover the blender with its lid and then pulse at high speed for 1 minute or more until

Watermelon Smoothie

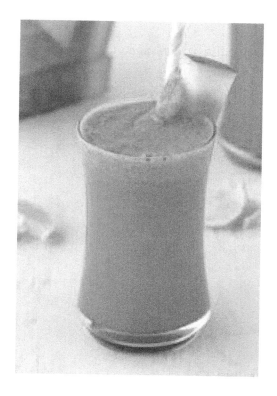

Preparation Time: 15 minutes

Cooking Time: 0 minutes

Serves: 1

Ingredients

4 cups watermelon, deseeded, cubed

4 key limes, juiced

4 cucumbers, deseeded, sliced

Instructions:

Take a high-powered blender, switch it on, and then place all the ingredients inside, in order.

Cover the blender with its lid and then pulse at high speed for 1 minute or more until

Lettuce and Orange Smoothie

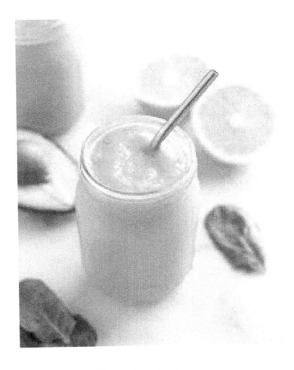

Preparation Time: 5 minutes

Cooking Time: 0 minutes

Serves: 2

Ingredients

1 cup coconut water

1 cup lettuce leaves, fresh

1 key lime, juiced

1 Seville orange, peeled

1 tablespoon bromide plus powder

½ of a medium avocado, pitted

Instructions:

Take a high-powered blender, switch it on, and then place all the ingredients inside, in order.

Cover the blender with its lid and then pulse at high speed for 1 minute or more until

Pear, Berries, and Quinoa Smoothie

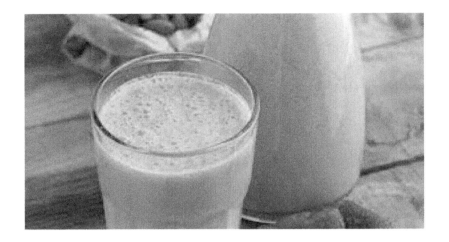

Preparation Time: 15 minutes

Cooking Time: 0 minutes

Serves: 1

Ingredients

2 cups spring water

½ of avocado, pitted

2 fresh pears, chopped

½ cup cooked quinoa

¼ cup fresh whole blueberries

Instructions:

Take a high-powered blender, switch it on, and then place all the ingredients inside, in order.

Cover the blender with its lid and then pulse at high speed for 1 minute or more until

Mango and Banana Smoothie

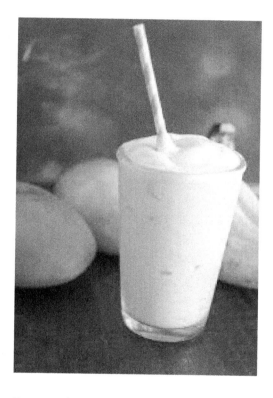

Preparation Time: 15 minutes

Cooking Time: 0 minutes

Serves: 1

Ingredients

1 cup spring water

2 cups greens

½ of banana, peeled

1 fresh mango, peeled, destoned, sliced

Instructions:

Take a high-powered blender, switch it on, and then place all the ingredients inside, in order.

Cover the blender with its lid and then pulse at high speed for 1 minute or more until

Toxin Flush Smoothie

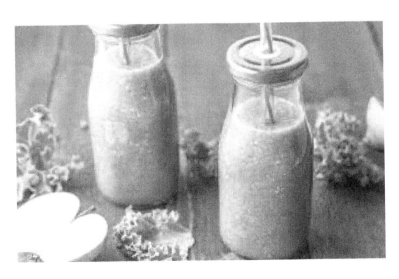

Preparation Time: 15 minutes

Cooking Time: 0 minutes

Serves: 1

Ingredients:

A key lime

A cucumber

Cubed, seeded watermelon, 1 c

Instructions:

Wash and dice the cucumber. Add the watermelon and cucumber to the blender and mix until combined. You shouldn't need to add extra water since both the watermelon and cucumber are mainly water.

Slice the lime in half and squeeze the juice into your smoothie. Enjoy.

Berry Peach Smoothie

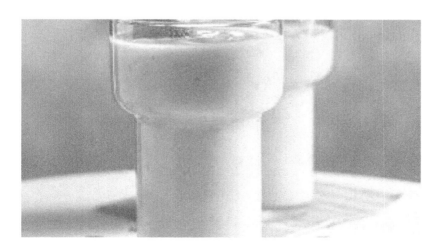

Preparation Time: 5 minutes
Cooking Time: 5 minutes

Serves: 2

Ingredients

1 cup coconut water

1 tbsp. hemp seeds

1 tbsp. agave

1/2 cup strawberries

1/2 cup blueberries

1/2 cup cherries

1/2 cup peaches

Instructions

Place all the ingredients into a blender then blend until they become smooth and creamy.

Serve.

Avocado Kale Smoothie

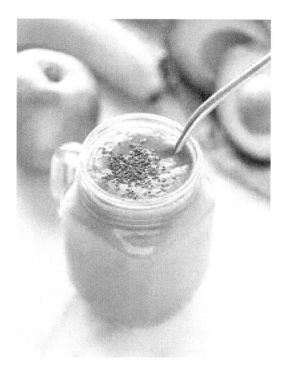

Preparation Time: 5 minutes

Cooking Time: 5 minutes

Serves: 3

Ingredients

1 cup water

1/2 peeled Seville orange

1 avocado

1 peeled cucumber

1 cup kale

1 cup ice cubes

Instructions

Place all the ingredients into a blender then process until they are smooth and creamy.

Serve and enjoy.

Apple Blueberry Smoothie

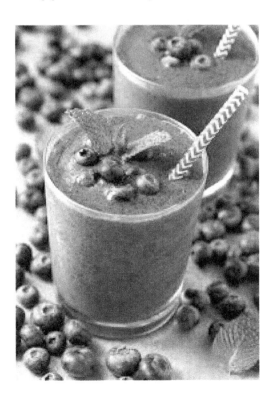

Preparation Time: 15 minutes

Cooking Time: 0 minutes

Serves: 1

Ingredients:

1/2 apple

1 Date

1/2 cup blueberries

1/2 cup sparkling callaloo

1 tbsp. hemp seeds

1 tbsp. sesame seeds

2 cups sparkling soft-jelly coconut water

1/2 tbsp. bromide plus powder

Instructions:

Mix all the ingredients in a high-speed blender.

Serve and enjoy!

Papaya Detox Smoothie

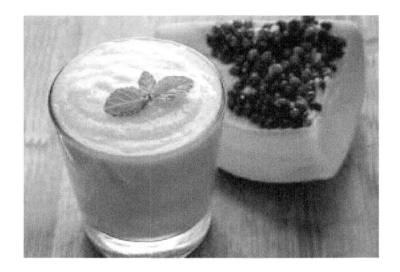

Preparation Time: 15 minutes

Cooking Time: 0 minutes

Serves: 1

Ingredients:

2 cups chopped Papaya into square pieces

1 tbsp. papaya seeds

Lime juice

1 cup filtered water

Instructions:

Place the ingredients into a high-speed blender then process for about 1 minute until all the ingredients are finely blended.

Serve and enjoy.

Chapter 18: 21 days meal plan and meal prep for rapid weight loss with Dr Sebi diet

DAYS	BREAKFAST	LUNCH/DINNER	SNACKS/DESSERT
1	Detox berry smoothie	Irish Sea Moss Alkaline Electric Recipe	Pumpkin Spice Crackers
2	Apple and amaranth detoxifying smoothie	Lasagna	Spicy Roasted Nuts
3	Arugula and Cucumber Smoothie	Kale and Brazil Nut Pesto with Butternut Squash	Potato Chips
4	Dandelion and Watercress Smoothie	Fried Rice	Zucchini Pepper Chips
5	Triple Berry Smoothie	Green Vegetable Diet	Onion Rings

6	Watermelon Smoothie	Taquitos Made with Mushroom	Flatbread Sloppy Joe
7	Lettuce and Orange Smoothie	Veggie Pizza	Apple Chips
8	Pear, Berries, and Quinoa Smoothie	Rice and Spinach Balls	Kale Crisps
9	Mango and Banana Smoothie	Roasted Vegetables	Zucchini Chips
10	Toxin Flush Smoothie	Curried Zucchini	Turnip Chips
11	Berry Peach Smoothie	Mushrooms and Rice	Blueberry Muffins
12	Avocado Kale Smoothie	Sautéed Radish	Baked Stuffed Pears

13	Apple Blueberry Smoothie	Tangy Lentil Soup	Dr. Sebi strawberry banana ice cream recipe
14	Papaya Detox Smoothie	Turnip Green Soup	Strawberry Sorbet
15	Respiratory Support Tea	Lentil Kale Soup	Banana Strawberry Ice Cream
16	Energizing Lemon Tea	Chive Celery Soup	Chocolate Pudding
17	Tranquil Tea	Pumpkin Squash Soup	Butternut Squash Pie
18	Date Syrup	Cauliflower Curry Soup	Cheesecake
19	Ginger Turmeric Tea	Zucchini Turnip Soup	Banana Cream Pie

20	Immune Tea	Soursop Ginger Soup	Homemade Whipped Cream
21	Mucus Cleanse Tea	Roasted Vegetable and Coconut Milk Soup	Alkaline-Electric Ice Cream

Conclusion

Dr. Sebi's diet is an entirely new approach to food. As such, it might be hard to get used to it, especially at the start.

It is advisable to try Dr. Sebi's method for 30 days if you do not fully adopt a new dietary regime. Engage for a month and see the improvements.

After a month, you might want to switch to this diet entirely. The next step is to start getting the supplements that you feel you should take. The great thing about picking out the supplements is that you can easily get help on the website to figure out which ones you need. Then you should start making changes to your diet. Even before you receive your Dr. Sebi products, you can go ahead and start following his nutritional guide. This is a big step in taking control of your health. While it may take a lot of changes, you can do it, and your body will thank you for it.

The Dr. Sebi Diabetes Cure can handiest work when finished nicely and with the proper herbs and the fine exceptional products. It is the truth that diabetic patients will go through issues and obstructions in their life because of their disease. However, with the right and proper care, their life would be revived. Consuming the right food and attaching yourself to the right diets will make you live your best life and make you healthy.

Dr. Sebi's alkaline diet is a popular diet made for curing illnesses that have been followed by many people. But scientific studies do not show that it results in curing any type of chronic disease. It is now seen as a method to lose weight and follow a healthy lifestyle to improve overall health.

It can provide all the benefits that a low calorie and high fresh vegetable and fruit diet can give. The benefits are enormous, but the level of calories should wander close to the calories you burn on average, or else you will feel lethargic, and a process called cell starvation will start. However, if your main goal is to reduce weight, it can give promising results.

Now, you have gotten hold of the information in this book. These Dr. Sebi approved information and tips will do you great good and benefits beyond your imagination and expectation. Good luck to everyone who has decided to embark on the journey of alkaline dieting! I hope that you carefully follow the Instructions: of this diet to get closer to your desires and healthy life

Made in the USA
Monee, IL
04 November 2020

46731926R00125